COMBAT FAT

FOR KIDS

The Complete Plan for Family Fitness, Nutrition, and Health

COMBAT FAT
FOR KIDS

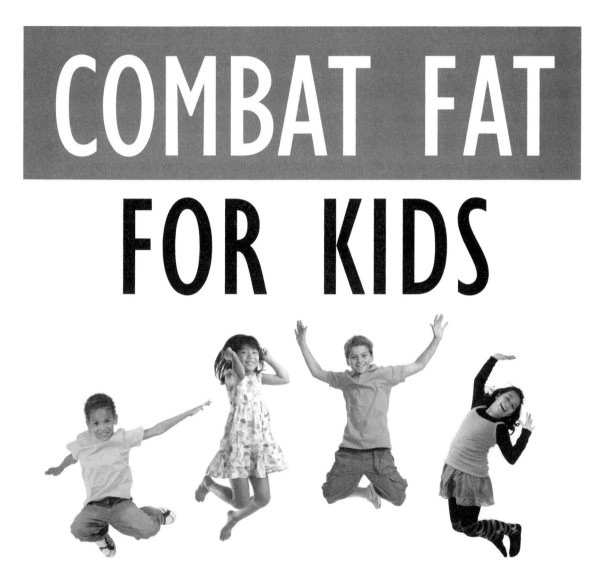

The Complete Plan for Family Fitness, Nutrition, and Health

JAMES VILLEPIGUE, CSCS **& JO BRIELYN**

Illustrations by Ariel Delacroix Dax

Foreword by Stuart Fischer, M.D.

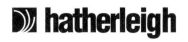 **hatherleigh**

Hatherleigh Press is committed to preserving and protecting the natural resources of the earth. Environmentally responsible and sustainable practices are embraced within the company's mission statement. Hatherleigh Press is a member of the Publishers Earth Alliance, committed to preserving and protecting the natural resources of the planet while developing a sustainable business model for the book publishing industry.

DISCLAIMER
This book does not give legal or medical advice. Always consult your doctor, lawyer, and other professionals. The ideas and suggestions contained in this book are not intended as a substitute for consulting with a physician. All matters regarding your health require medical supervision.

Library of Congress Cataloging-in-Publication Data is available.
ISBN: 978-1-57826-**396-7**

All Hatherleigh Press titles are available for bulk purchase, special promotions, and premiums. For information about reselling and special purchase opportunities, please call 1-800-528-2550 and ask for the Special Sales Manager.

Cover Design by Dede Cummings Designs
Interior Design by Dede Cummings Designs
Illustrations by Ariel Delacroix Dax

Printed in the United States

10 9 8 7 6 5 4 3 2 1

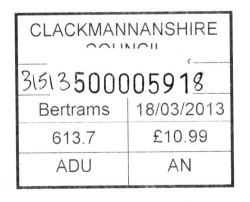

CONTENTS •••••••••••••••••••

Foreword by Stuart Fischer, M.D. vii
Introduction 1

PART I   THE CYCLE OF OBESITY 5

Chapter 1 • **Causes of Obesity** 7

Chapter 2 • **Common Challenges to Staying Fit as a Family** 17

PART II   DIET AND NUTRITION 29

Chapter 3 • **Nutrition Basics for Healthy, Active Kids** 31

Chapter 4 • **Family-Friendly Meal Plans** 53
           • Parent-Prepared Meals 62
           • Kid Creations 113

Chapter 5 • **Tips on Eating at Home and Dining Out** 123

PART III EXERCISE   133

Chapter 6 • **Fitness Basics for Healthy, Active Kids** 135

Chapter 7 • **Easy Does It! (Fun Timed Activities)** 147

Chapter 8 • **Get Out and Play! (Outdoor Recreational Activities)** .. 175

           FAQ's 187
           Resources 191

FOREWORD $\bullet \bullet \bullet \bullet \bullet \bullet \bullet \bullet \bullet \bullet \bullet \bullet \bullet \bullet \bullet \bullet \bullet$

by Stuart Fischer, M.D.

EPIDEMIC CHILDHOOD OBESITY IS a health crisis with potentially more disastrous consequences than any other challenge the United States faces at the present time. Despite advances in medical technology and emergency care, the next generation of Americans has a shorter life expectancy than their parents, a troublesome statistic unprecedented in recorded history. Obesity is a risk factor for 40 different illnesses in nine different organ systems including diabetes, hypertension, even asthma and mood disorders.

Parents have long sought a comprehensive yet enjoyable plan of action, one that develops lifelong health priorities and self-control as part of their children's education. Without good health, their journey into the future may have significant obstacles, impediments that can be avoided only by early intervention. The solution requires proper caloric balance, regular exercise, avoidance of peer-pressure, development of self-confidence, and multiple other important life lessons.

Such a solution is superbly delineated in this excellent book, which is an indispensable addition to every parent's library. Mothers and fathers have always been the ideal life-coaches, and their role in treating and preventing obesity cannot be duplicated by any government, insurance, or scholastic program. *Combat Fat for Kids*, superbly and engagingly written by James Villepigue and Jo Brielyn, belongs in your home. The rewards of better health and a longer lifespan are priceless.

STUART FISCHER, M.D., a graduate of Yale University, completed his residency at Maimonides Hospital in Brooklyn, and served as an Attending Physician at Cabrini Medical Center in New York City. He also worked with the late Dr. Robert Atkins as the Associate Medical Director of the Atkins Center. His expertise in alternative medicine, nutrition, and weight loss, is complemented by his strong traditional, hospital-based education. He is author of *The Park Avenue Diet* and *The Little Book of Big Medical Emergencies*.

INTRODUCTION · · · · · · · · · · · · · · · · · · ·

H EY, KIDS AND FAMILIES! Welcome to *Combat Fat for Kids!* Thanks for letting us come into your homes and lives to shake up things. Today—this very moment—is the time to make a change for the better. We know you agree. That's the reason you opened this book and why we're about to embark on a life-changing journey together!

The state of fitness in our nation has changed over time and the way families view fitness must adjust with it. The health of our children and future generations depends on it. Childhood obesity is a dangerous epidemic that is on the rise in our country. There is a genuine need for adults and kids to learn how to make wiser decisions regarding nutrition and exercise and to implement those solutions into their daily lifestyles. The fact that you've selected *Combat Fat for Kids!* and are ready to make healthy decisions indicates your awareness that change needs to happen in our country and in your own home.

Let us first state that *Combat Fat for Kids!* is more than just a book. Often when we read a book, we nod our heads in agreement, remark to ourselves or to someone close by that it was indeed a "good book," and then tuck it away on a shelf and forget about it. In this case, however, we encourage you to view this less as a book and more as a plan of action to kick-start and guide your family on your journey toward healthier lifestyles.

Sure, the first time you flip through the pages, we suggest that you read it straight through to the end, as you would a typical book. Many of your questions will be answered and concerns addressed simply by reading the information we have provided for you. It will also help you get a better overall understanding of the obesity issue, how the *Combat Fat for Kids!* approach works, and how it applies to your own family. However, our challenge to you is to take it a step further once you've read the book, and start to implement changes in your home.

Don't limit your interaction with *Combat Fat for Kids!* to a one-time reading from beginning to end. Feel free to jump around the book any way you please. If you're struggling with the exercise portion or need to spice up your current routine, read the last chapters first. When you need inspiration for new meals, go straight to the recipes. The content is available any way you need it and is yours for the taking.

Our vision in creating *Combat Fat for Kids!* is to provide a simple, effective plan and tool that kids and their families can use on an ongoing basis. We understand that your family approach will fluctuate and grow as your kids do. This means that sometimes your needs and concerns will change, or new questions may arise. Keep this book close by and refer to it often.

KEEP F.U.N. AT THE CENTER

The *Combat Fat for Kids!* program has three main principles that lead to its success for children and their families. We selected the acronym FUN to identify them because we believe that fun should be included in every nutritional and exercise program, especially one geared toward families and kids. After all, what kid (or parent) doesn't want to have fun? Fun motivates, keeps excitement alive, and makes eating smart and exercising regularly seem less like work and more like simply the best choice for living life well.

* Fitness
* Understanding
* Nutrition

Fitness: Families will find easy-to-follow instructions and suggestions for incorporating fitness and activity into their daily routines in the fitness portion of this book. The pages of this section are filled with fun and effective activities, from more structured activities and exercises to inventive free play games for kids and their parents to enjoy together.

Understanding: Understanding remains at the core of the program. Sandwiched between the fitness and nutritional aspects of our program is the need for knowledge and understanding. In order for parents, kids, and families to gain the full benefits of *Combat Fat for Kids!* they need to know why it's necessary, how it works, and tricks for how to keep the momentum alive in their family.

Nutrition: The nutrition section provides everything from explanations of nutrition basics to suggestions on how to plan and shop for your family's meals, all the way to creative tricks to use when introducing new, healthier foods into your child's diet. You will also find a large variety of delicious, nutritious recipes for you and your family. There's even a section devoted to our young budding chefs that contains healthy and easy-to-make recipes for kids to make on their own or with their parents.

UNDERSTANDING THE SYMBOLS AND SECTIONS

We've designed this book with all of our readers in mind, both adults and kids. Here are a few symbols that you will see used throughout to make it easier to identify sections that might be of special interest.

⭐ *Tips from the top!* These sections offer practical advice and tips from noted experts in the fields of fitness and nutrition.

⭐ ⚡Quick Drill When you see these areas, take 10 to 20 minutes and complete the action or exercise with your family.

⭐ Psst . . . Parents Some material is meant strictly for parents' eyes. This symbol is your indicator.

⭐ 💡Think About It The Think About It sections are designedto give you a thought or principle to consider and reflect on. Allow yourself to be challenged by these!

⭐ ⚙ KIDS' CORNER We have not forgotten the sources of our inspiration for this book: the kids. Kids' Corner segments are our opportunity to talk directly to your kids and encourage them.

GET READY, GET SET, AND GO!

We commend you for taking the first step toward improving the overall health of your kids and family by picking up *Combat Fat for Kids!* Now it's time to put action to that good intention and get into the battle. Remember to work hard, stick together as a family, and have FUN while doing it. You have *Combat Fat for Kids!* in your hands, so you're already set. Now get ready and go!

PART I

THE CYCLE OF OBESITY

Chapter 1

CAUSES OF OBESITY • • • • • • • • • •

A S PARENTS AND CAREGIVERS, we all want to see children living happy and healthy lives. Yet, the reality is statistics have proven that kids today are not healthier than in years past. In fact, a greater number of them are inactive, out of shape, fighting illnesses related to their lack of fitness, and in the end, traveling down the road toward a long battle with obesity. The obesity rate for kids in the United States has tripled in the past 30 years. The youth of today have an expected life span that is less than that of their parents!

We don't present these facts to condemn anyone or to promote a sense of hopelessness—our goal is just the opposite. The driving purposes behind *Combat Fat for Kids!* are to educate, empower, and call families to action.

It's time to face the truth. There is a disconnect happening somewhere between that dream we have for our kids and the reality that is hitting American children and their families today. But the important thing to remember is that change *is* possible. Although it is going to take more than dreams to make the change, this book will show you how to implement action—with kids, schools, parents, and entire families!

So, before we dive into how to make changes for your kids and your family, let's get a better picture of how obesity is currently affecting American youth and their families.

THE HARD-HITTING FACTS

* Data from the 2007–2008 National Health and Nutrition Examination Survey (NHANES) concluded that approximately 12.5 million American children and adolescents between the ages of 2 and 19 are obese.

✳ About 17% of all children and adolescents in the United States today are obese. That's 1 out of every 6 kids! An additional 15% of American youth are overweight.

✳ The percentage of children 6 to 11 years old in America who were obese increased from 7% in 1980 to nearly 20% in 2008. Over the same time period, the percentage of youth 12 to 19 years old who were obese increased from 5% to 18%.

✳ In 2008, over one-third of all adolescents were considered overweight or obese.

✳ Kids and adolescents that are obese have increased risk factors for developing cardiovascular diseases, like high blood pressure and high cholesterol.

✳ Obese youth are at greater risk for sleep apnea, diabetes, joint and bone issues, and social and psychological problems such as low self-esteem and discrimination.

✳ Children and teenagers who are obese are more likely to become obese adults, making them more susceptible to a slew of diseases that have been linked to adult obesity: stroke, heart disease, type 2 diabetes, osteoarthritis, and several types of cancer (including cancer of the kidney, pancreas, breasts, colon, prostate, cervix, ovary, endometrium, esophagus, gall bladder, and thyroid).

HOW CAN I TELL IF MY CHILD IS OVERWEIGHT OR OBESE?

First of all, let's define what the difference is between being overweight and obese. Both are terms used for weight ranges that are higher than what is generally considered healthy for a particular height. Overweight is defined as having, for a given height, excess body *weight* that comes from a combination of fat, muscle, water, and bones. Obesity refers to having excess body *fat* for a given height.

The American Academy of Pediatrics (AAP) and the Centers for Disease Control and Prevention (CDC) have both recommended the Body Mass Index (often referred to as BMI) to screen for overweight and obesity in youth between the ages of 2 and 19. BMI is a useful method in assessing whether or not a person is at a healthy weight, or is underweight, overweight, or obese. Consulting the BMI chart (see pages 10 and 11) can help you make a quick determination as to whether or not your child may have a weight issue. When doing so, keep in mind that BMI also has limitations. The Body Mass Index is not a diagnostic tool, and the BMI chart does not clearly differentiate between fat and muscle. For example, individuals with a higher muscle mass, such as athletes, may have a higher BMI but, in fact, still be at a healthy weight.

BMI is calculated using a formula that is based on the ratio of weight to height squared. Unlike the BMI chart for adults, age and sex are also factors when determining body mass for children and adolescents. This is necessary because the amount of body fat changes with age. The healthy range of body fat also differs for boys and girls.

$$BMI* = [weight / (height \times height)] \times 703$$

This formula uses weight in pounds and height in inches.

Underweight: BMI that is less than the 5th percentile refers to being underweight.

Healthy weight: BMI that is from the 5th percentile up to the 85th percentile indicates a healthy weight.

Overweight: BMI that is from the 85th up to 95th percentile refers to being overweight.

Obese: BMI that is equal to or greater than the 95th percentile refers to being obese.

CDC Growth Charts: United States

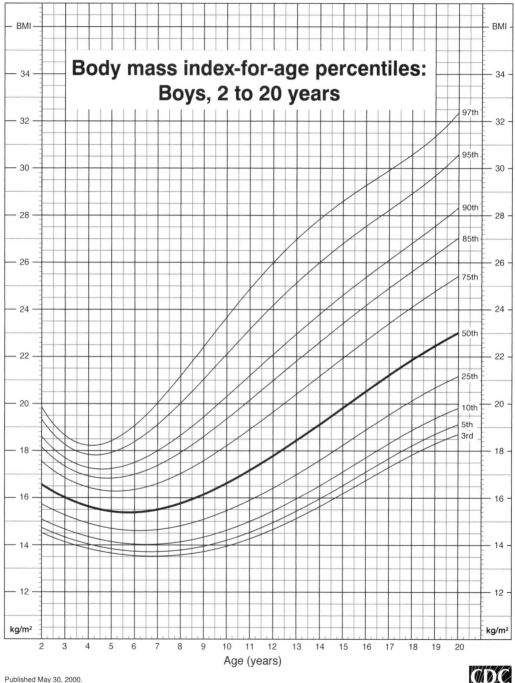

Body mass index-for-age percentiles:
Boys, 2 to 20 years

Published May 30, 2000.
SOURCE: Developed by the National Center for Health Statistics in collaboration with
the National Center for Chronic Disease Prevention and Health Promotion (2000).

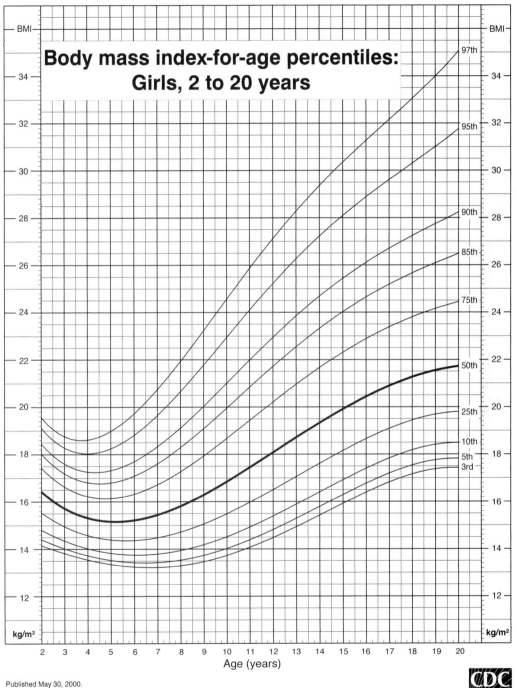

Body mass index-for-age percentiles: Girls, 2 to 20 years

BMI

97th
95th
90th
85th
75th
50th
25th
10th
5th
3rd

Age (years)

kg/m²

Published May 30, 2000.
SOURCE: Developed by the National Center for Health Statistics in collaboration with
the National Center for Chronic Disease Prevention and Health Promotion (2000).

SAFER · HEALTHIER · PEOPLE™

A visit to your family physician may also provide a clearer answer of whether or not your child has a weight problem. She or he can perform further assessments, such as skinfold thickness measurements, health screenings, examination of the child's diet and activity level, and a closer look at the family history.

Tips from the top!

"Obesity is a family illness," says Debra Haire-Joshu, PhD, principal investigator and director of the Obesity Prevention Center at Saint Louis University School of Public Health. "Children typically are not born obese. They learn to become obese in an environment that encourages it. If parents are eating poorly, that's what they're providing their children."

—"'Obesity is a family illness;' research offers clues on how to stop the cycle." *Obesity, Fitness & Wellness Week,* July 5, 2003: 24. *Health Reference Center Academic.*

CAUSES OF WEIGHT PROBLEMS

Overweight and obesity are both products of an imbalance of energy in a person's body. Simply put, they are the result of eating too many calories and not getting enough physical activity. A *calorie* is a unit of energy that is supplied by food or drinks. Regardless of what kids are eating and drinking, they are still accumulating those calories. Calories themselves are not a bad thing; the body needs calories. It's the imbalance of calories that causes weight problems. The child's body uses some of those calories in everyday bodily functions; then the excess calories are burned through physical activity and exercise. To maintain a caloric balance, and therefore maintain a healthy body weight, there needs to be a balanced relationship between the number of calories consumed and the number of calories burned. If kids are consuming calories and not burning them through an active lifestyle, they end up with an overabundance of calories. That excess is what leads to overweight and obesity.

Environment, metabolism, and genetic factors may also affect a person's weight gain, but the diet and physical activities a child or adolescent chooses make a huge difference in his or her likelihood of becoming overweight or obese.

Genetics and the Childhood Obesity Epidemic

Do genetics play a part in the childhood obesity epidemic? Sure they do, but the genetic role does not account for the majority of the problem. Over the span of the last 30 years, the childhood obesity rate in our nation has more than tripled. If genetics were the driving force behind that rise in obesity, how can it be explained that the offspring of the same adults who were kids 30 years ago have a much higher rate of obesity than their parents did as children?

Although it may not be the primary factor, the genetic background of a child does play some role in his or her likelihood to become overweight or obese. Genetics determine not only body type but also how the body stores and burns fat. In some cases, genes may increase a kid's susceptibility for obesity, but genes do not necessarily predict a future of obesity. Genetics alone do not sentence a child or adult to such a life. Changing outside behavior factors, like poor food choices or lack of physical activity, can greatly counteract a genetic disposition to weight gain and obesity.

We know more than ever before about the damaging effects of living an unhealthy lifestyle but the statistics cannot be denied. This question begs to be answered: Why, in the most progressive age for information and technology, are children and families facing the highest obesity rate in history?

Technology

Ironically, instead of facilitating a positive change, technology often plays an adverse role in the fight against childhood obesity. The youth of today are inundated with technology that offers time-wasting, sedentary forms of entertainment. Television, video games, movies, computers, the Internet, and cellular phones with texting capabilities are all excellent inventions when used in moderation. Too often, though, lounging around the house playing with these gadgets replaces other, more physical, activities like riding bikes and playing sports.

Statistics provided by Let's Move! (a comprehensive initiative launched by First Lady Michelle Obama in 2010 that is dedicated to solving the problem of childhood obesity) show that 8- to 18-year-old kids spend an average of 7.5 hours each day using entertainment media like television, video games, cell phones, computers, and movies. That means approximately half of the hours that America's youth are awake each day are filled by using technology! Data also concludes that only one-third of high school students in the United States engage in even the minimum amount of recommended physical activity each day.

What does that tell us? It's time to get off the couch and find active forms of entertainment!

Tips from the top!

"Despite obesity having strong genetic determinants, the genetic composition of the population does not change rapidly. Therefore, the large increase in . . . [obesity] must reflect major changes in non-genetic factors."

—Hill, James O., and Frederick L. Trowbridge, "Childhood obesity: Future directions and research priorities," *Pediatrics*, 1998; Supplement: 571.

Our Schools

Twenty to 30 years ago, kids walked to and from school every day, ran around at recess, and participated regularly in gym class and extracurricular sports. In the interest of saving time and money, carpools and bus rides have replaced the morning and afternoon walks, recess is often left out to accommodate busy class schedules, and physical education classes and after-school sports programs are being cut. All of this means that, during the school day, kids are not getting as much physical activity as in past years.

In addition, the food that children consume while at school is an increasing problem. Walk into almost any American school cafeteria today and take a look at what is being served to kids. School menus now more closely resemble a fast food restaurant than a healthy, home-cooked meal. Items like pizza, burgers, fries, and processed chicken nuggets are the typical fare served in our schools every day. And if those types of meals weren't causing enough harm to the diets of our children, vending machines stocked with sodas and junk food are now commonplace in many schools. But don't lose hope yet. There are some great initiatives taking place in schools across the United States, many of them student-driven. We'll tell you more about them in chapter 3 and in the Resources section.

Processed and Fast Foods

The desire for convenience has become one of the leading criteria for food choices in America today. More families are buying processed, ready-to-eat meals to prepare at home or eating fast food or restaurant meals. According to a new survey conducted by the Institute of Food Technologists, "less than a third of Americans are cooking their evening dinners from scratch. Although 75% of Americans claim to eat dinners at home, almost half those meals are fast food, delivery, or takeout from restaurants or grocery delis." For the most part, children now eat more meals that are not home-cooked, drink more sugar-sweetened and caffeinated drinks, and snack more often. The majority of those foods are consumed on the go, without much thought as to how much fat, sugar, salt, additives, and calories are entering the body with every bite.

And let's not discount the overwhelming lure from restaurants to "king-size" those already calorie- and fat-laden portions! Did you know that portion sizes in restaurants grew between 1977 and 1996? The average portion sizes for salty snacks increased from 1.0 ounce in 1977 to 1.6 ounces in 1996. Soft drinks grew from an average serving of 12.2 ounces in 1977 to a whopping 19.9 ounces in 1996.

So at the same time that our kids are spending less time doing physical activities, they're also consuming more calories by eating fatty, packaged foods.

Stress (for Parents and Kids)

As we mentioned previously, a fast-paced lifestyle and the desire for immediate results permeates most of American life today. A great majority of parents work long hours to pay the bills and struggle to find time to care for the needs of their family. When you add in duties like chauffeuring kids to and from activities and school, shopping for necessities, and running errands, family members often find they are spending more time in the car than in their own home. In a fast-paced environment such as this, stress levels are sure to be high. Financial stresses, relationship stresses, parenting stresses, work stresses, health stresses . . . the list goes on and on. Kids certainly aren't immune to this, either. The truth is, when one member of the family is stressed, the whole family feels it. So how does stress factor in to the rise in obesity?

People who are stressed often make poor food decisions and reach for comfort foods, which are usually high in sugar or fats. Interestingly enough, researchers have found proof that the body releases specific hormones that boost this action. When an individual eats carbohydrates, the body creates more serotonin. Serotonin is the feel-good chemical for the body, so when someone is stressed they tend to reach for carbohydrate-heavy foods to self-medicate. Studies have also shown that chronic stress causes the body to produce an excess of cortisol, which is a hormone that manages energy use and fat storage. Cortisol may also increase appetite and cravings for fatty or sugary foods. George Chrousos, MD, Chief of the Pediatric and Reproductive Endocrinology Branch at the National Institute of Child Health and Human Development (NICHD), and Philip Gold, MD, Chief of the Clinical Neuroendocrinology Branch at the National Institute of Mental Health (NIMH) concluded in their report in 2002 that stress can increase appetite and lead to weight gain. Stress further stimulates obesity by releasing a molecule called neuropeptide Y (NPY) that unlocks fat cells in the body and causes them to increase in size and number.

The good news is there are a number of stress-relieving activities you and your kids can practice to reduce daily stress and relax together.

A FAMILY NEED FOR MORE EDUCATION ON HEALTHY LIVING

When an individual is overweight or obese and fails to lose weight, it is sometimes thought to be due to a lack of motivation or self-control from her or him. Actually, the problem is often due more to a lack of health education, especially for children and teenagers. The desire to lose weight and live a healthier life may be there, but it can be difficult to achieve positive results without the knowledge of how to make healthy choices.

It's not just kids who need more education on making healthier food and fitness decisions. Many parents were never taught how to properly make those choices, either. That's where *Combat Fat for Kids!* comes in. When you're done reading this book, you and your whole family will have the knowledge necessary to create and keep a healthy lifestyle . . . and have fun together while doing it!

Chapter 2

COMMON CHALLENGES TO STAYING FIT AS A FAMILY • • • • •

YOU NOW UNDERSTAND HOW serious childhood obesity is and are ready to make healthy lifestyle changes when *wham!* reality sets in and hits you dead on with the challenge of making those changes mesh with real life. Yes, it's a given: challenges will come, especially when you're striving to make major adjustments in your family members' lives and routines. Change is not easy for anyone, and kids are certainly no exception. We're parents too and we understand that. We face the same challenges with our own children and families!

But don't walk away from the battle just yet. The journey is only just beginning and the rewards of fit kids and a healthier family are worth the effort. Your best defense against life's challenges is to recognize them and learn ways to combat them. So, pick up your weapons and get ready to combat fat!

THE TIME CRUNCH

One of the greatest challenges faced by families today is the lack of time to accomplish all they need, or want, to do each day. There just don't seem to be enough hours in the day. When time is compressed, it is often things we consider to be *extras* that are pushed aside. Taking care of our bodies and fueling them with the proper foods should be our primary concern, not the last, but that is often not the way things play out. For many, physical activity and mealtime become afterthoughts when schedules are busy.

In fact, there are people who may be busier than you and yet are still out there exercising and eating right. So how do they do it? They make a conscious effort.

They plan and prepare beforehand. They prioritize and make time for it. They also understand that missing one day due to time constraints doesn't mean giving up the whole effort. It simply means you'll need to jump back into the routine tomorrow.

Planning and enlisting time-saving strategies may seem impossible when your schedule is already strained, but these techniques will save you and your family time in the long run.

Tips from the top!

"Although it takes time to implement healthy lifestyle habits, the return on investment is tremendous—which makes the time investment worth it. Another helpful item is to look at managing weight not as something 'extra' to do, but rather a part of our everyday lifestyle. Just as we eat and sleep every day, we should get some type of physical activity every day, whether it's exercise, activities throughout the day or both."

—Donald Hensrud, MD. "Tips to save time, eat healthy and exercise regularly." Mayo Clinic. July 10, 2012. http://www.mayoclinic.com/health/healthy-lifestyle-tips/

Here are a few time-saving ideas to try with your family:

★ *Make planning meals a family effort and plan your meal calendar in advance.* The purpose of a meal calendar is to serve as a guideline, so there's still some room for flexibility if plans change or you decide to swap a meal with another one on the list. Create your meal schedule and post it in the kitchen where the whole family can see it. This will save you time—and money—when you grocery shop by providing a detailed plan that you can stick to. It will also help keep eating healthier meals on task and eliminate the last-minute run for fast food because a meal went unplanned for. Also, allowing kids to be involved in the planning will teach them valuable skills about how to plan balanced meals and make wiser food decisions.

★ *Designate a Saturday or Sunday as cooking day and enlist the help of the entire family.* Prepare several healthy meals in advance and use a vacuum sealer to preserve and freeze the meals in proper portion sizes. Cooking in advance will save you hours of prep time during the week and will make it possible for you to still serve the family a well-balanced meal on those busy evenings.

* *Make healthy snack alternatives readily available to your kids.* Part of the appeal of prepackaged snack items is that they are easy to grab and go. Utilize this same principle when offering your kids healthy choices. Use resealable bags or containers to measure out your own single-serving packages of nuts, seeds, and other healthy snack alternatives. Wash and chop vegetables and fruits before storing and keep them on a shelf in the refrigerator where the whole family can reach them.

* *Make a decision as a family to cut out one unnecessary sedentary activity and replace it with a more active choice of entertainment.* For instance, instead of sitting down to watch a television show after dinner, use that same 60 minutes to take a family bike ride or play outside together. You just made time to exercise together without giving up anything of true significance!

⚡ QUICK DRILL

(Take 20 minutes and do this now!)

Sit down with your kids and make a quick list of what you believe are the challenges your family will face in the journey to combat fat together. Write down every answer that is given. You are not limited to only the challenges listed in this chapter; we have only covered a few common challenges that families may face. Don't question someone's suggestion and don't argue about it. Just because one member doesn't see an issue as a challenge doesn't mean it is not a true obstacle for someone else. If it's a challenge for one member, it's a challenge for the whole family. Once your list is complete, go back and discuss each one in more detail. Come up with at least one positive response your family will make to overcome each obstacle. Post your list of challenges and solutions in a central place for your family so you can refer back to it later. *Remember, you are a team and you're in this together!*

THE BATTLE OF THE JUNK FOOD LOVERS AND PICKY EATERS

If mealtime and snack time often result in struggles to get your children to eat healthier foods, don't lose hope. You are not alone! In fact, most parents will agree that having a child who always wants to eat healthy foods is quite rare.

Whether your child is a junk food lover or a picky eater, the struggle is equally as challenging. Some days, it can be tempting to give in and buy that greasy burger and fries or to serve macaroni and cheese for the third night in a row simply so your child will eat something. The dinner table often becomes a battleground between parents and children. After a busy day, few parents want to deal with a power struggle over who is eating their vegetables and who isn't. Getting kids—and the whole family, for that matter—to eat more nutritious meals doesn't have to be a constant battle. Some creativity and flexibility will go a long way in bridging that gap.

Try these tips to help ease junk food lovers and picky eaters into a healthier diet:

* *Begin by mixing healthier elements into foods that your child already likes.* For instance, if your child loves to eat pancakes, toss some fresh blueberries or strawberries into the batter next time you prepare them. Does your kid like rice? Shred some carrot or squash on top of the rice before serving it.

* *Let them dip the healthy foods in something.* Kids simply find dunking food fun! When you serve meat or vegetables to your child, provide ketchup, cottage cheese, hummus, or a homemade dipping sauce on the side. Be forewarned: their choice of dipping sauces may not always look appealing to you, and there will be more potential for messes, but the pros outweigh the cons on this one, so take the chance!

* *Help kids to make better choices by keeping junk food out of the house and having healthier choices close by.* If kids are hungry for a snack, they are going to grab what's quick and available to them. Keep junk food and processed snacks on the store shelves, not in your cupboards. Instead, stock up on healthier choices like yogurt, cheese, fruits, and vegetables, and store them in a place that is easy for kids to access. You may be surprised to see that your junk food

lovers and picky eaters will start to make wiser food choices on their own once they get into the habit at home. That doesn't mean kids won't ever choose to eat junk, especially when they are away from home, but they will put more thought into their decision and will be less likely to choose those items.

* *Don't push too hard if your child doesn't like something.* It's wise to offer a wide selection of foods for kids to try so they can discover which ones they like the best. If (or when) you encounter foods that your child strongly dislikes, try not to make a big deal out of it. Instead, acknowledge that she or he was open to sampling it and move on. Be willing to provide a different healthy food as a substitute instead of pressuring her or him to force down something that she or he has tried and sincerely doesn't like. As long as he is eating a nutritious alternative, there is no reason to create a stigma for him about eating a certain food. In time, he may be willing to try it again and change his mind.

* *Get rid of the "clean your plate" rule.* Kids can tell when they feel full. It is not necessary to force them to eat when they feel stuffed simply because there is still food on the plate. One of the main reasons people, kids included, consume too many calories is because we tend to overeat. In fact, many adults who struggle with eating issues today can think back to their own childhood and remember sitting at the table forcing down every last morsel on their plates. Instead, encourage your child to eat enough to satisfy his or her hunger and then set the plate aside. Kids need to learn portion control at home.

* *Schedule snack time and stick to the routine.* Even healthy snacks should be monitored. We've all heard the story of someone eating an entire box of cookies and trying to justify it because they were fat-free. Just because foods are labeled as being good for you doesn't mean they can't still be culprits in the obesity problem if large quantities are consumed. Also, eating too many snacks may interfere with how well your child eats at mealtime. If kids know they are only allowed to eat at certain times, they will be more willing to eat what they are given when it is provided.

* *Introduce fun and lots of color to healthy foods.* Who says eating healthy can't be fun, too? Kids like variety, color, and fun, so use that to your advantage

when making them snacks and meals. Try lightening up dinnertime by hosting a color-coordinated night where all the foods you eat are green, orange, or whatever your child's favorite color is. Or, mix things up a bit and serve your child's typical sandwich in a tortilla or arrange her cut vegetables into the design of a flower or her favorite animal. The options are as vast as your imagination!

★ *Set the example.* Don't expect your kids to jump up and down with excitement when it's time to eat their broccoli if you won't even touch the stuff yourself. Kids watch everything we do, so parents *must* lead by example. The best way to help them learn healthy eating habits is to practice them in your own life.

THE THREE B'S FOR COMBATING FAT FOR KIDS!

★ *Be a role model for your child.* Living a healthier lifestyle is not about being perfect all the time. It's about doing your best to live a healthy life and letting your kids see that. It's even okay for them to see you fail occasionally, as long as you get back on track.

★ *Be positive, be positive, be positive!* Kids don't like to be told what they *can't* do—nobody does. Instead, focus on what they *can* do and what they are already doing well. Acknowledge areas that need improvement, but be liberal with your praise and encouragement and try to keep the main emphasis on their successes.

★ *Be realistic.* Remember, the goal is not perfection! The ultimate goal is to make smarter choices for your family and to teach them how to make healthy decisions for themselves.

TECHNOLOGY—FRIEND OR FOE?

Technology itself isn't a bad thing. On the contrary, technology has produced many discoveries that make our lives and jobs safer and more efficient, and make life easier every day. Unfortunately, it has also introduced a wide variety of distractions into our homes that were not there even 30 or 40 years ago. It is now more uncommon to hear of families who *don't* have television sets, computers, video games, and cellular phones than to meet those who *do* own them. In many cases, there are even multiple TVs and other electronic devices in the household. Truthfully, there is nothing wrong with using these devices—in moderation. The trouble comes into play when using these devices, most of which require the users to remain sedentary for long periods of time, begins to take the place of living more physically active lives.

Technology is only going to expand as new developments are made, so the key to success is to learn how to take advantage of technology in moderation and to use it for our family's benefit instead of detriment.

Try these tips for starters:

* *Save vegging out for at the dinner table, not in front of the TV or computer!* Eating in front of the computer or television is distracting and may cause kids to develop poor eating habits. Also, it's much easier to overeat when you're busy watching a show instead of paying attention to how much you're eating.

* *Set a limit on how many hours a day family members will have screen time— whether in front of the television, on the computer, or playing video games— and stick to it.*

* *Try substituting one hour of active entertainment for one hour of your family's typical inactive entertainment every day.* Simply put, skip one television show and spend that time being active together!

🔆 Think About It
The Importance of Communication

What you say to kids and how you say it makes a huge difference in how they look at themselves. Yes, they need you to be direct about the importance of their health. They also need you to remember that they are still developing their body image and self-esteem. And regardless of what they may lead you to believe at times, your opinion does matter to them!

Fitness expert James Villepigue knows firsthand the impact an adult's words and actions can have on a child struggling with weight issues. Think about this:

"Adults aren't always the best support. I'll never forget the day when I was in the nurse's office—the school nurse also happened to be my mom—during my junior high school days. The football coach happened to stroll in and he looked me up and down. He then told me to follow him. My first thought was that he wanted to recruit me for the team. I followed him back into the gym storage room. A big old scale stood in the back of the room. He told me to get on and he began moving the balance rods back and forth. His hand came to a stop and he looked up at me and said, "Do you see this? You are 255 pounds. Look what you did to yourself!" That's all he said, and all he ever said to me ever again.

I was humiliated and became very depressed by that episode. If anything, it sent me spiraling downward. This was the moment in my life where a single person who I actually looked up to could have helped me, but rather, he hurt me and casually created my new identity.

Prior to this incident, I was not depressed or self-conscious. I had so much love from family and friends, and even though I may have been made fun of by my peers, I had never yet experienced abuse from an adult . . . from someone who I looked up to and respected and the source of critical feedback that mattered most! That man was, in his own way, trying to help me, not hurt me. That moment has been forever imprinted on my mind—I can remember the incident vividly as if it has just happened. That's pure emotional pain and it could have been prevented if that teacher had only known how to guide a child."

THE SKINNY ON BODY IMAGE

Self-esteem and body image play a significant role in the lives of kids of all ages, but it can be especially challenging when they hit adolescence. Kids are always under pressure to fit a certain image. The mold changes with time, but the pressure remains the same. Children and adolescents are bombarded with images on TV, on the Internet, and in magazines that depict what a so-called perfect guy or girl should look like. They compare themselves to an airbrushed and skewed standard that is unrealistic, and quite frankly, often dangerous for them to try to attain.

Here are some tips to encourage a positive body image for your kids:

* *Work on building and maintaining a stronger relationship with your child.* All youth will battle some level of confidence issues, but a tighter bond with a parent, close family member, or guardian can help boost self-esteem.

* *Reassure your kid often.* Help her or him focus on their strengths, not their flaws. Adolescents, in particular, often dwell on being too tall or too short, how much acne they have, and how they think their body should measure up to those of their peers. With all of this negativity, it can be easy for them to forget all the wonderful things about themselves. We sometimes get caught up in the same cycle, even as adults.

* *Be open about any weight issues you feel your child—and you—may have but remember to deal with them tactfully.* We're not saying to tiptoe around the problem or pretend it doesn't exist. Just the opposite! Your kid needs you to face the issues head on, but remain clear that being overweight or obese does not define the person. Reinforce this point often.

* *Talk frankly to your kids and explain that being a certain size does not mean a person is healthy.* There are many unhealthy ways to lose weight that are not good for the body, some are even dangerous. Be sure to explain to your kids how they can get fit in a healthy way.

* *Awareness is important.* Be aware of what your kids are eating, how often they are eating, and how much they are eating. Awareness must go beyond watching their food habits, though. Pay attention to drastic changes in your child's

behavior, energy levels, performance at school or home, and health. These may be signs that something more serious is going on with your child.

Psst . . . Parents

Watch for Dangerous Eating Habits

Unhealthy eating habits can make children and adults sick and can be lethal without intervention. Eating disorders are a very real problem and no one is immune. Boys and girls, kids and adults can all develop eating disorders. Awareness is the best protection against them.

THE MOST COMMON PITFALLS

Here are the most common eating disorders, along with the basic signs to look for:

Anorexia

An individual with anorexia, or anorexia nervosa, has an intense fear of gaining weight. She or he usually severely limits food intake and often becomes dangerously thin.

A few signs of anorexia include:

* losing a lot of weight
* denying being hungry (even if they are)
* exercising too much
* feeling fat or always complaining about being fat
* withdrawing from social activities
* loss of menstrual period in girls or women of ovulation age

Bulimia

Instead of starving himself or herself, a person with bulimia will binge and purge. A bulimic will eat large quantities of food (usually unhealthy items like junk food), and then vomit or use laxatives to eliminate the food from the body. Kids and adults who suffer from bulimia often see this as a way to control what they eat, and by extension, to control their lives.

A few common signs of bulimia include:

* eating large quantities of food without weight gain
* making excuses to go to the bathroom immediately after eating meals
* withdrawing from social activities
* hiding food and food wrappers in the bedroom
* using laxatives, diuretics, or diet pills

Binge Eating or Compulsive Overeating

Unlike with bulimia, someone who binge eats gorges on large amounts of food but will not usually purge afterward. Compulsive eating is generally categorized by impulsive or continuous eating beyond the point of comfort.

A few common signs of compulsive overeating include:

* eating excessive quantities of food on impulse
* dieting or fasting sporadically
* exhibiting signs of anxiety, depression, self-hatred, or loneliness
* having a body weight that ranges from normal to varying levels of obesity

If you believe that you or your child is suffering from an eating disorder, please seek medical attention immediately. Eating disorders can cause damage to vital organs in the body, such as the heart, liver, and kidneys, and can also cause psychological harm.

For more information, you can speak with the operators at the National Eating Disorders Association (NEDA) Helpline at (800) 931-2237.

SIMPLE WAYS TO LEND POSITIVE SUPPORT AND ENCOURAGEMENT TO KIDS

* *Set your child up for success.* Make healthy choices readily available and teach her or him how to judge correct portion sizes. This empowers the child to be healthy on his own and lessens the need for you to constantly remind him, an approach that many kids see as nagging.

* *Avoid trying to scare kids healthy.* We're all for being direct with kids about the seriousness of getting and staying healthy. They need to know the truth and hear it straight. What we're against is the use of tactics that bully or demean the child. This type of approach can backfire and affect the emotional health of the child. Angst-ridden kids often become depressed or anxious and turn to food for comfort.

* *Choose words that build up the child, not belittle her or him.* Cutesy pet names and teasing may seem harmless to adults, but if they focus on a kid's body image, they won't seem harmless to the child. For instance, a dad might think that calling his overweight son "Slim" is humorous and he may mean no ill intent by it. Yet the child may fail to see the humor in that and can view the name as more hurtful than funny. Stick with nicknames and comments that uplift, not ones that pinpoint a child's faults!

* *Get involved with your child and have fun doing it!* The best way you can encourage and lend support to a child who is trying to get healthier is to make your efforts a family affair. Don't make them just about his or her need to get in shape. Instead, focus on the whole family getting fit and healthy together. Plan and prepare tasty, healthy meals together. Find family activities that get you moving as a group and make getting fit a fun adventure instead of a chore.

PART II

DIET AND NUTRITION

Chapter 3

NUTRITION BASICS FOR HEALTHY, ACTIVE KIDS • • • • • • •

A HEALTHY AND BALANCED DIET helps kids grow stronger, live longer, and learn better. Practicing proper nutrition also helps prevent childhood obesity and reduces the risks of developing weight-related diseases like diabetes and high blood pressure. A healthy diet also stabilizes moods and sharpens children's minds. If you begin teaching and encouraging healthy eating habits for your child now, you can make a big impact on their lifelong relationship with food, offering them the opportunity to grow into strong, health-conscious adults.

> The health and safety of your kids are important to you—and to us. That's why credibility is so crucial in this nutrition section. The nutritional information provided in this book is based on the 2010 Dietary Guidelines for Americans, the Centers for Disease Control and Prevention (CDC), the United States Department of Health, and the American Academy of Pediatrics.

You won't find any radical eating programs or fad diets suggested here. There are no quick, easy fixes to childhood obesity. Diet trends and fads may cause an initial weight loss and excitement, but they do not last. The answer to overcoming the battle with fat is not found in a trendy program. We believe in making smart and safe lifestyle changes that will benefit your kids today and for the rest of their lives. The *Combat Fat for Kids!* approach to nutrition and fitness promotes education, finding a healthy balance, and making wiser choices as a family.

Let's begin with a few basics about nutrition.

WHAT ARE CALORIES?

"Don't eat that! It has too many calories in it." You have most likely heard someone say this before, but what exactly does it mean? Are calories bad for your child?

A calorie is a unit of measurement, but interestingly enough, even though the term is usually associated with weight gain it doesn't actually measure weight or size. A calorie is a unit of energy and the calories found in an item measure how much energy the body gets from eating or drinking it.

Calories aren't bad for your child. It isn't the consumption of calories that leads to weight gain or obesity. In fact, calories sustain your child's body and stamina. The body requires them for energy. Bodily functions such as breathing and the heart pumping blood cannot even happen without an adequate supply of calories. A child's growing body also needs the energy that calories provide in order to mature and develop. The real culprit for weight gain is consuming more calories than the body needs and not burning off the excess ones through physical activity. As a result, leftover calories convert to fat in the body, and excess body fat leads to obesity. The solution is learning how to find foods and drinks that offer a good mix of nutritional value along with necessary calories, instead of consuming empty calories. We'll get into that in more detail later in this chapter.

How Many Calories Should My Child Consume?

Not all children are created the same size and every person's body burns energy—and calories—at a different rate, so there isn't an exact number of calories that all kids should consume. Most school-age kids require between 1,600 and 2,200 calories a day, depending on their age, activity level, and gender. For example, a child who participates in athletics or is more physically active than his or her peers may need to consume extra calories. Caloric requirements also increase during puberty, so it is important to keep that in mind as your child grows and matures.

DAILY ESTIMATED CALORIES FOR KIDS
According to Age and Gender

Child's Age	Daily Estimated Calories
1 Year	900 Calories (both girls and boys)
2–3 Years	1,000 Calories (both girls and boys)
4–8 Years	1,200 Calories (girls) / 1,400 Calories (boys)
9–13 Years	1,600 Calories (girls) / 1,800 Calories (boys)
14–18 Years	1,800 Calories (girls) / 2,200 Calories (boys)

Please note that these calorie estimates are based on a child with an inactive lifestyle. When a child increases his or her physical activity, more calories will be required. If the child is moderately active, 0 to 200 calories should be added. If she or he is extremely physically active, add another 200 to 400 calories to the daily diet.

⚡ QUICK DRILL

FOOD LABELS AND CALORIES

Calories are listed on food labels by serving size, and serving sizes for foods vary a lot according to the product. When you start reading food labels, you will be surprised by some of the serving sizes. For instance, a quick look on the grocery shelf will prove that a serving size for one box of multigrain crackers may only be three crackers, while another type of multigrain cracker may allow as many as nine crackers per serving—that's a significant difference!

In order to calculate the number of calories your child is getting, you will need to:

1. Find the serving size at the top of the food label.

2. Determine how many calories are in one serving.

3. Decide how many servings your child is going to consume.

4. Multiply the number of calories for one serving size by the number of servings she or he eats to find the total calories.

Let's return to our example with the wheat crackers for a moment. The box lists three crackers as a serving size. If your child chooses to eat six crackers, she or he is really eating two servings, not one. If there are 70 calories per serving size and he eats two servings, you must double the number of calories to determine the correct amount of calories being consumed. In this case, he is actually eating 140 Calories.

Make this calorie calculation into a game with your school-age child by having him help figure out the answer. Not only is it a great opportunity to practice math skills, but he'll also be learning how to eat smarter and will be taking an active part in his own health!

CONSIDER THE ONE-THIRDS APPROACH TO DIET

⅓ fat + ⅓ protein + ⅓ carbohydrates = 1 healthy kid

As we mentioned at the beginning of this chapter, the *Combat Fat for Kids!* approach focuses on finding a healthy balance for your kids and your whole family. It's an approach that doesn't simply refer to the need for balance between nutrition, physical activity, and rest. It also applies to your daily food intake! Your child's diet should consist of approximately one-third dietary fat, one-third protein, and one-third carbohydrates. It is recommended that between 25% and 35% of an average kid's daily diet should be made up of dietary fat. Another 25% to 30% is usually derived from protein. About 45% of the daily intake for kids is typically recommended to be from carbohydrates. While the intake of carbohydrates is slightly above the one-third mark, remember that the one-thirds concept will make it easier for you to find a healthy balance in your family's diet.

> This approach is based on the premise that your child has no preexisting illnesses or special dietary needs. If your child has any special dietary needs or requires a strict diet plan, please consult your pediatrician or dietician to determine the eating approach that best fits his or her specific health needs.

Students Cook up Change
for Nutritious School Lunches

In 2007, the Healthy Schools Campaign (HSC) launched Cooking up Change in Chicago and involved student chefs and the community in talks about the need for food reform in the nation's school systems.

Now, HSC is the driving force behind the Cooking up Change initiative and works with local sponsors in cities across America to host qualifying contests. The contest challenges student chefs to come up with a delicious school lunch that also meets nutrition standards—while adhering to a tight budget and using only the ingredients typically available to school food service workers.

Teams from six cities met the challenge in the 2011–2012 contest season. Local competitions for students studying culinary arts were held in Chicago, Denver, Jacksonville, Santa Ana, St. Louis, and Winston-Salem. The winning teams from each of those cities then represented their home city and battled it out in the national finals in May 2012.

Want to learn more about how these students are transforming the look and recipes of schools across America or want to learn how to get involved with the Cooking up Change initiative? Visit the event page on the Healthy Schools Campaign's website: www.healthyschoolscampaign.org/event/cookingupchange/2012/natl/index.php

WHAT IS DIETARY FAT?

Not all fat is bad. In fact, your child's body needs fat to function correctly. Fat serves as a great source of energy to the body and also helps it absorb vitamins. An adequate amount of fat is also necessary for your child to grow and develop. There are, however, some fats that are better than others.

Try to limit these fats in your child's diet:

* *Saturated fats*: Saturated fats come primarily from animal sources like dairy and meat products and occur naturally in many foods. Foods that are high in saturated fat also often increase cholesterol in the blood, which contributes to clogged arteries that block the flow of oxygen-rich blood to the brain and heart. Some examples of foods and drinks that contain saturated fats are poultry with the skin, pork, fatty beef, butter, solid shortening, lard, cream, cheese, and other dairy products made from whole or reduced-fat milk. A lot of fried foods and baked goods also have high levels of saturated fats.

* *Trans fats*: Trans fats (also called partially hydrogenated oils) are fats that are man-made in factories to make vegetable oils more solid by adding hydrogen to liquid vegetable oil. Trans fats raise the LDL (low-density lipoprotein) cholesterol level, or "bad" cholesterol level, in the body, increasing your child's risk of heart disease. Trans fats are found in many packaged snack foods, cookies, crackers, vegetable shortenings, some margarines, fried foods like doughnuts and French fries, and baked goods like pizza dough, biscuits, pastries, and pie crusts.

Try to replace saturated and trans fats with polyunsaturated and monounsaturated fats. These are better choices for fat and can be found in oils like canola oil, soybean oil, olive oil, and sunflower oil. Other sources of these "good fats" include many nuts and seeds, avocados, peanut butter, and fatty fish such as salmon, trout, and mackerel.

Polyunsaturated fats: Polyunsaturated fats contain more than one double-bonded (unsaturated) carbon in the molecule. What does that mean for your child? In moderation, polyunsaturated fats reduce cholesterol levels and lower the risk of developing heart disease. They also provide the body with the essential fats—omega-3 and omega-6—that it doesn't naturally produce. Both omega-3 and omega-6 play an important role in brain function and in the daily growth and development of your child's body.

Monounsaturated fats: Monounsaturated fats have one double-bonded (unsaturated) carbon in the molecule, but unlike polyunsaturated fats that remain in a liquid form, monounsaturated fats are generally liquid at room temperature but begin to change to solid when chilled. Much like polyunsaturated fats, they reduce cholesterol levels and lower the risk of developing heart disease. They also provide your child's body with nutrients that develop and maintain body cells and are high in vitamin E, an antioxidant that helps maintain a healthy immunity system and is believed to protect against cancer and heart disease. Some examples of foods that are high in monounsaturated fats include vegetable oils (such as olive oil, canola oil, peanut oil, sunflower oil, and sesame oil) as well as avocados, peanut butter, and many nuts and seeds.

Tips from the top!

"Parents play a critical role at home in preventing childhood obesity, with their role changing at different stages of their child's development. By better understanding their own role in influencing their child's dietary practices, physical activity, sedentary behaviors, and ultimately weight status, parents can learn how to create a healthful nutrition environment in their home, provide opportunities for physical activity, discourage sedentary behaviors such as TV viewing, and serve as role models themselves."

—Gortmaker, Steven, et al. "The role of parents in preventing childhood obesity." The Future of Children," Spring 2006: 169+. Health Reference Center Academic.

WHAT IS PROTEIN?

Every tissue, cell, and organ in your child's body is made of protein. Protein is necessary for building and repairing body tissues, creating energy and stamina, and making hormones and enzymes that the body uses for a number of processes. The body's proteins are constantly being used, so there is always a need for them to be replaced by new ones. Protein that is found in the food and drink your child consumes is digested into amino acids, which band together like building blocks and are later used to replace the proteins in the body.

Protein is found in the following foods:

* Eggs
* Nuts
* Seeds
* Meats, poultry, and fish
* Legumes (dry beans and peas)
* Tofu
* Milk and dairy products
* Grains
* Some vegetables and fruits (such as apricots, tomatoes, broccoli, and lettuce)

Animal-based foods (like meat, poultry, fish, milk, eggs, and cheese) are considered complete protein sources because they provide the body with all of the essential amino acids.

How Sweet Are Your Child's Food and Drink Choices?

Typically, foods and drinks that contain added sugars have fewer nutrients than foods that have naturally occurring sugars. A good way to limit added sugars for your child is to read the ingredients list on food labels and know what you're looking for. Sugar additives come in many forms, so simply looking for the word "sugar" is not enough.

Whenever you see any of the items listed below on a product's ingredients list, it means that the food or drink contains added sugars. The closer the ingredient is to the top of the list, the more of that sugar is found in the food. If more than one of these sugar additives is listed, the item has an even higher level of sugar in it.

All of these ingredients are forms of added sugars:

* Sugar
* Syrup
* Sucrose
* Raw sugar
* Molasses
* Corn syrup
* Malt syrup
* High-fructose corn syrup
* Brown sugar

* Corn sweetener
* Honey
* Fruit juice concentrates
* Invert sugar
* Dextrose
* Lactose
* Maltose
* Fructose
* Glucose

WHAT ARE CARBOHYDRATES?

Carbohydrates (or carbs) are sugars and starches that break down in your child's body to provide energy.

Carbohydrates can be found in:

* Vegetables
* Fruits
* Breads and other grains
* Milk and dairy products
* Foods that have added sugars (such as sugar-sweetened drinks, cookies, and cakes)

There are two basic types of carbohydrates: simple carbohydrates and complex carbohydrates.

Simple Carbohydrates

Simple carbohydrates are sugars that are found naturally in foods like vegetables, fruits, milk, and dairy products. They are generally easier for the body to digest and can be used up by the body for quick energy. Simple carbohydrates may also be found in foods that are processed and refined like pasta, white sugar, and white bread.

Complex Carbohydrates

Complex carbohydrates are sugars that are found naturally in foods like vegetables, whole grain breads and pasta, brown rice, and legumes. Complex carbohydrates take longer for the body to digest. Foods that have unrefined grains (like brown rice) preserve those complex carbohydrates better than refined grains (like white rice) because the refining process takes away some of the natural fiber and nutrients of the grain. So eating a serving of a complex carbohydrate will fill your child up and provide energy longer than eating a serving of a simple carbohydrate or sugary choice.

There are two forms of complex carbohydrates: starch and dietary fiber.

Starch is found in vegetables like potatoes, peas, and dry beans. It is also found in some breads and grains. The body breaks down starch when it digests it and uses it as a source of glucose, which provides energy.

Dietary fiber is found mainly in fruits, vegetables, whole grains, and legumes. It consists of all the parts of plant-based foods that the human body does not absorb or digest. Your child's body digests other food components (like fats, proteins, and simple carbohydrates), but it doesn't digest fiber. Instead, fiber travels through the body mostly intact. Yet it still aids in bowel functions, lowers cholesterol, helps regulate sugar levels, and helps with weight loss.

Fiber is also classified into two categories: those that don't dissolve in water (insoluble fiber) and those that do (soluble fiber). Soluble and insoluble fibers affect the human body in different ways, but both are beneficial. Soluble fiber dissolves in water inside the small intestine, which helps slow down digestion. In addition, when soluble fiber attaches to cholesterol in the body, it prevents the body from absorbing the cholesterol and helps reduce cholesterol levels. Unlike soluble fiber, insoluble fiber does not dissolve in water. Since it cannot be absorbed by the intestines, insoluble fiber usually passes through the digestive system quickly. Insoluble fiber also helps other foods in the body to pass through the digestive tract quicker, which results in more bowel movements and less constipation.

> Many foods that derive from plants, like seeds and fruits, contain both soluble and insoluble fiber. Include food items that contain both types of fiber in your child's daily diet.

Some sources of insoluble fiber are:

* Whole-wheat bread
* Brown rice
* Barley
* Couscous

* Seeds
* Most vegetables
* Fruits

A few sources of soluble fiber are:

* Nuts
* Seeds
* Oatmeal

* Most fruits (such as pears, apples, strawberries, and blueberries)
* Dry beans and peas

How Whole Are Your Child's Grain Choices?

Whole grains are an excellent source of fiber and nutrients. The term "whole grain" applies to grains that still have all three parts of the grain seed or kernel (bran, germ, and endosperm). The Dietary Guidelines for Americans recommends that at least half of the daily fiber choices for your child should be from whole grains. So, when you look at the food label, how do you know if the product contains whole grains?

Here are some ways that whole grains may be listed:

* Whole-grain barley
* Whole-grain corn
* Whole oats (oatmeal)
* Whole rye
* Whole wheat
* Brown rice

* Wild rice
* Bulgur (cracked wheat)
* Buckwheat
* Millet
* Quinoa
* Triticale

THE FIVE MAIN FOOD GROUPS

Most adults who grew up in the United States are familiar with the United States Department of Agriculture's (USDA) Food Guide Pyramid with its six vertical stripes representing five food groups plus oils. In 2011, the USDA unveiled a new, easier to understand symbol to help Americans remember to eat healthy: MyPlate.

MyPlate, an icon that looks like a cup and dinner plate with dividers, illustrates the five food groups that are the building blocks for a healthy diet. The plate displays four sections: vegetables, fruits, grains, and protein. The cup in the icon represents the dairy, such as a cup of milk, although those dairy servings can also come from yogurt or cheese.

The MyPlate model can be used for breakfast, lunch, and dinner. While all breakfasts may not include vegetables, the aim should be to include a fair blend of food groups with every meal.

If your child's breakfast doesn't include a vegetable, try serving a vegetable at snack time. The MyPlate image serves as a helpful reminder that your family should eat a variety of foods while also aiming to eat less of unhealthy food types (such as junk food, items with sugar additives, and foods that contain saturated and trans fats).

Drinking Smarter!

★ *Add a twist to water and make it more exciting!* Try adding a slice of lemon, lime, berries, or another favorite fruit to your child's ice water.

★ *Mix up H$_2$O drinks by combining water or sparkling water with a splash of 100% juice.*

★ *When water is cold and available, kids will reach for it more often.* Buy each member of the family a special reusable water bottle, keep the bottles refilled and chilled when not in use, and carry them with you when you go out for the day.

★ *If your child does choose to indulge in a soda or sugary drink, encourage her or him to choose a smaller size than normal.*

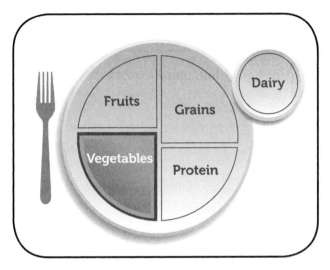

Courtesy of ChooseMyPlate.gov

Common Sources for Vegetables

Any food that is a vegetable or 100% vegetable juice is considered a member of the Vegetable Group. They may be fresh, frozen, or canned and can be served either cooked or raw. The USDA recommends that half of your child's plate be filled with vegetables and fruits.

* Dark green vegetables (like broccoli, kale, romaine lettuce, and spinach)
* Starchy vegetables (such as corn, plantains, green peas, and potatoes)
* Red and orange vegetables (like butternut squash, carrots, red peppers, sweet potatoes, and tomatoes)
* Beans and peas (such as black beans, garbanzo beans, kidney beans, lentils, and white beans)
* Other vegetables (like avocado, beets, cabbage, green peppers, mushrooms, and zucchini)

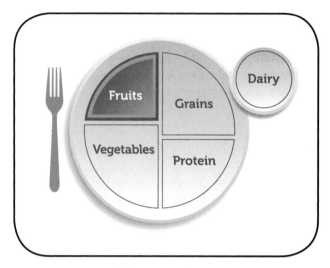

Courtesy of ChooseMyPlate.gov

Common Sources for Fruits

Any food that is a fruit or 100% fruit juice is a part of the Fruit Group. They may be fresh, frozen, canned, or dried. The USDA recommends that half of your child's plate be filled with vegetables and fruits.

* Apples   * Raisins

* Cherries   * Berries

* Grapefruit   * Melons

* Oranges   * 100% fruit juices

* Plums

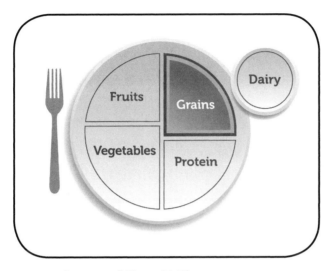

Courtesy of ChooseMyPlate.gov

Common Sources for Grains

Food made from wheat, rice, oats, cornmeal, barley, or another cereal grain are considered part of the Grain Group. The recommended amount of grain for a child each day depends on his or her age. The USDA recommends that children 2 to 3 years old consume 3 one-ounce equivalents of grain, kids ages 4 to 8 should receive 5 one-ounce equivalents, girls ages 9 to 13 should get 5 one-ounce equivalents, girls ages 14 to 18 need 6 one-ounce grain equivalents, boys ages 9 to 13 should consume 6 one-ounce equivalents, and boys that are 14 to 18 need 8 one-ounce equivalents. At least half of the child's daily grain intake should be whole grains.

* Bread
* Pasta
* Rice
* Oatmeal

* Tortillas
* Grits
* Flour

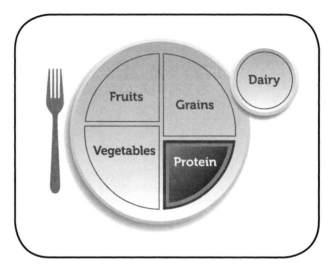

Courtesy of ChooseMyPlate.gov

Common Sources for Protein

Foods that come from meat, poultry, seafood, beans and peas, eggs, processed soy products, nuts, and seeds are considered part of the Protein Group (you may notice that beans and peas are also part of the Vegetable Group). The recommended amount of protein for a child each day is dependent upon their age, as well as gender. The USDA suggests that children 2 to 3 years old have 2 one-ounce equivalents each day, kids ages 4 to 8 get 4 one-ounce equivalents, girls ages 9 to 18 years old consume 5 one-ounce protein equivalents, boys 9 to 13 get 5 one-ounce equivalents, and boys ages 14 to 18 years old, 6 ½ one-ounce equivalents of protein daily.

- ⋆ Whole meats and ground meats (such as lean cuts of beef, ham, lamb, pork, and venison)
- ⋆ Organ meats (like liver and giblets)
- ⋆ Poultry (such as chicken, turkey, goose, duck, and ground turkey and chicken)
- ⋆ Eggs
- ⋆ Beans and peas (like black beans, lima beans, navy beans, soy beans, and pinto beans)
- ⋆ Processed soy products (such as tofu, veggie burgers, and tempeh)

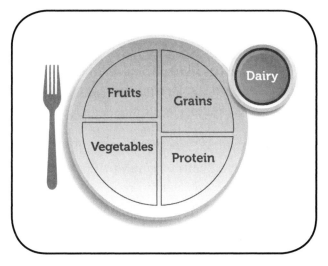

Courtesy of ChooseMyPlate.gov

Common Sources for Dairy

Milk and foods that are made from milk and that retain their calcium content are part of the Dairy Group. Foods that are made from milk but have little or no calcium content (like cream cheese or butter) are not included in this group. Children should consume 2 to 3 cups of dairy each day, so try to include 1 cup of dairy with each meal.

★ Fluid milk (including skim, low-fat, reduced-fat, whole milk, flavored milks, and lactose-free or lactose–reduced milks)

★ Calcium-fortified soymilk

★ Cheese (like cheddar, mozzarella, Swiss, American, ricotta, and cottage cheese)

★ Yogurt (including fat-free, low-fat, reduced-fat, and whole milk yogurts)

★ Milk-based desserts (such as ice cream, frozen yogurt, and pudding)

Psst . . .   Parents

Hydrate: Meeting Your Child's Daily Water Needs

Think about how droopy your flowers look when you forget to give them water for a day or two. Remember how they perked back up after you gave them some water? That same concept applies to humans. Yet, paying attention to our kids' water intake is something many of us parents forget to do on a daily basis. Staying hydrated is a crucial step in your family's journey to a healthier lifestyle.

Water is not only good for your child's body, it's essential to it. Water helps regulate body temperature by ridding the body of excess heat through sweat. It also lubricates joints, aids in digestion, carries nutrients to body cells, rids the body of wastes, is essential for muscle structure and function, and provides needed moisture to the respiratory system. Water flows throughout your child's entire body and makes up about 75% of his body weight.

Essentially, it is recommended that your child consume two to three quarts of water in a day (about eight to twelve 8-ounce glasses of water). The majority of your child's water needs will most likely be met through the water and beverages she or he drinks. However, some foods, such as soup broth and some vegetables and fruits, contain water (tomatoes, celery, oranges, and melons all consist of almost 85 to 95% water). A good way to sneak in most of those daily doses of water is to encourage kids to drink one glass of water with each meal and a glass of water in between each meal, such as at snack time.

It is also important to make sure that your child drinks water before she or he even feels thirsty. Thirst is a sign that the body is already in a state of dehydration.

Your child's body will also need higher quantities of water when she or he is:

* More physically active
* In a hot climate
* Sick with a fever, diarrhea, or vomiting

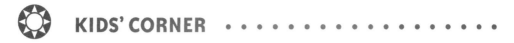

KIDS' CORNER

Hey, kids! Do you know that you can take an active part in controlling your own health by learning portion control? Portion control, what's that?

Well, a portion is how much you eat or drink of something. The truth is that most of our portions are much bigger than what we should be eating, so we're all getting extra calories that our bodies don't need. Look below for tips on learning to estimate healthy portions on your plate.

Here are some easy ways to estimate a healthy portion size:

* ✳ 2 to 3 ounces of meat, fish, poultry (approximately the size of a deck of cards)
* ✳ ½ cup rice or pasta (cooked)
* ✳ 1 cup milk or yogurt
* ✳ ¾ cup fruit juice
* ✳ 1 slice of bread
* ✳ 2 ounces cheese (about the size of a domino)
* ✳ 1 small piece of fruit (larger pieces of fruit are 2 or more servings)
* ✳ ¼ cup dried fruit
* ✳ ½ cup grapes (about 15 of them)
* ✳ 1 egg
* ✳ 1 ½ cups ice cream
* ✳ 1 tablespoon peanut butter
* ✳ 1 teaspoon butter or margarine (about the size of a postage stamp)
* ✳ 1 ounce chocolate

Make sure to ask your parent or another adult to show you how to use measuring cups and spoons for your food, too. You can, and should, help keep track of your portions!

Making a slight change in the size of your portions can make a huge difference in getting healthy. Next time before your meal or snack, take a look at the food and drink in front of you. How do your portions measure up to the guides above?

Chapter 4

FAMILY-FRIENDLY
MEAL PLANS • • • • • • • • • • • • • •

W E UNDERSTAND THAT PLANNING healthy family meals and snacks may seem like a daunting task, especially if you're new to it. Keep in mind that variety and flexibility are the keys to success for getting kids to eat healthier meals. These same approaches work well for adults, too!

To get you started on your journey to making healthier food choices, we have created a sample meal plan for you to follow. This meal plan will also serve as a guideline when you begin planning your own family meals. In the following pages, you will find choices for every meal, plus a snack, for an entire week. We have also included 50 healthy and delicious recipes for your family to enjoy.

We encourage you to involve your kids in the preparation and cooking of these family recipes so they can learn healthy cooking methods. We've also included 10 healthy and tasty recipes in the Kid's Creation section (page 113) for kids to make themselves. Responsible kids ages 10 and up should be able to prepare these recipes alone, but we do recommend adult supervision and a quick lesson on kitchen safety—such as how to clean foods, handle knives, and use the microwave. Younger children will be able to help with simpler portions of the recipes but some adult participation will still be necessary.

Make Your Choice!

To use the choices provided on the next few pages:

* Select one meal from the **BREAKFAST** choices (page 55).

* Choose one meal from the **LUNCH** choices (page 57).

* Take your pick from the **DINNER** choices (page 59).

* For snacks, make your selections from the **SNACK** choices, typically one to two snacks per day (page 61).

When making your meal choices for the day, keep in mind the daily caloric requirements for each family member, and be sure to maintain a proper balance of all the food groups mentioned in Chapter 3 (page 44). Remember, kids of different ages, gender, or activity level may not require the same amount of calories as other family members. We advise serving the same meals for your whole family, but you may need to slightly alter the portion sizes for some family members.

COMBAT FAT FOR KIDS! BREAKFAST CHOICES

Breakfast Choice #1

1 Breakfast Fruit Wrap (page 121)
1 cup milk
1 eight-ounce glass of water

Breakfast Choice #2

1 Banana Oatmeal Muffin (page 66)
1 small orange
1 cup milk
1 eight-ounce glass of water

Breakfast Choice #3

1 Red and Yellow Pepper Omelets (page 69)
1 banana
1 cup 100% fruit juice
1 eight-ounce glass of water

Breakfast Choice #4

1 Breakfast Banana Smoothie (page 71)
2 slices whole-grain toast with 2 teaspoons peanut butter
1 eight-ounce glass of water

Breakfast Choice #5

1 bowl of Golden Apple Oatmeal (page 73)
1 small (1.5 oz.) box of raisins
1 cup milk
1 eight-ounce glass of water

Breakfast Choice #6

1 (6 oz.) low-fat yogurt mixed with 2 tablespoons Maple Raisin Granola
(page 74)
1 cup 100% fruit juice
1 eight-ounce glass of water

Breakfast Choice #7

1 Broccoli Frittata (page 70)
1 slice whole-grain toast with 1 teaspoon butter
1 eight-ounce glass of water

COMBAT FAT FOR KIDS! LUNCH CHOICES

Lunch Choice #1

1 bowl of Modified Macaroni 'n Cheese (page 75)
1 handful raw baby carrots
1 cup apple slices
1 eight-ounce glass of water

Lunch Choice #2

1 Apple Tuna Sandwich (page 76)
1 handful cucumber slices
1 handful pretzels
1 eight-ounce glass of water

Lunch Choice #3

1 Red, White, and Green Grilled Cheese sandwich (page 77)
½ bowl of Old-Fashioned Tomato Soup (page 83)
1 eight-ounce glass of water

Lunch Choice #4

1 Pita Pizza (page 80)
1 cup grapes
1 eight-ounce glass of water

Lunch Choice #5

1 bowl of Tuscan Chickpea Soup (page 81)
4 saltine crackers
½ plate green salad with low-fat dressing
1 eight-ounce glass of water

Lunch Choice #6

1 Turkey, Spinach and Apple Wrap (page 122)
¼ cup Spiced Toasted Almonds (page 103)
1 eight-ounce glass of water

Lunch Choice #7

1 Cheesy Cone (page 119)
1 handful cherry tomatoes
1 handful pretzels
1 eight-ounce glass of water

COMBAT FAT FOR KIDS! DINNER CHOICES

Dinner Choice #1

1 Chicken Quesadilla (page 87) with ½ cup Red and Green Salsa (page 87)
¼ plate brown rice
½ plate grilled vegetables
1 eight-ounce glass of water

Dinner Choice #2

¼ plate Orzo Skillet (page 89)
1 small vegetable salad with low-fat dressing
1 piece corn on the cob
1 eight-ounce glass of water

Dinner Choice #3

1 Smoky Mustard-Maple Salmon fillet (page 93)
¼ plate rice pilaf
1 cup Confetti Appleslaw (page 85)
1 cup steamed broccoli and carrots
1 eight-ounce glass of water

Dinner Choice #4

¼ plate Sweet and Sour Pork (page 96)
¼ plate brown rice
½ plate Outtasight Salad (page 86)
1 eight-ounce glass of water

Dinner Choice #5

¼ plate whole-wheat spaghetti topped with Super Meatballs with Spicy
    Red Sauce (page 91)
1 small whole-wheat roll
½ plate vegetable salad with low-fat dressing
1 eight-ounce glass of water

Dinner Choice #6

3 ounces Cornbread-Crusted Turkey with 1 cup carrots and sauce mixture
    (page 100)
1 small baked sweet potato
½ plate green salad with low-fat dressing
1 eight-ounce glass of water

Dinner Choice #7

2 slices of Garden Turkey Meatloaf (page 94)
1 small baked potato
1 small plate vegetable salad with low-fat dressing
1 small whole-wheat roll
1 eight-ounce glass of water

COMBAT FAT FOR KIDS! SNACK CHOICES

Snack Choice #1

1 handful Toasted Whole-Wheat Pita Wedges (page 104)
Chickpea Dip (page 107)

Snack Choice #2

1 Papaya Boats (page 109)

Snack Choice #3

1 Black Bean Brownie (page 112)

Snack Choice #4

1 Frozen Fruit Cup (page 113)

Snack Choice #5

1 Yogurt Parfait (page 116)
½ cup Maple Raisin Granola (page 74)

Snack Choice #6

1 Peanut Butter Quesadilla (page 120)

Snack Choice #7

1 Cheesy Cone (page 119)

oatmeal pancakes with cranberries

(Courtesy of American Institute for Cancer Research, www.aicr.org)

Serves 5

½ cup all-purpose flour
¼ cup whole-wheat flour
¼ teaspoon salt
1 tablespoon sugar
½ teaspoon baking powder
¾ teaspoon baking soda
¾ cup quick-cooking (not instant) oats
1 cup plain low-fat yogurt
1 cup low-fat milk
1 teaspoon vanilla extract
2 tablespoons canola oil
2 egg whites, lightly beaten
½ cup dried cranberries
Juice of 1 lemon (optional)
Canola oil spray, as needed

➤ Preheat the oven to 200°F. In a medium bowl, sift together all-purpose and whole-wheat flours. Add the remaining dry ingredients and mix well.

In a separate bowl, beat the yogurt, milk, vanilla, oil, and egg whites. Add the wet ingredients to the dry ingredients, making sure not to overmix. Stir in the cranberries. For the very best results, allow the batter to rest, covered, in the refrigerator for 30 minutes.

Spray a griddle or large, flat pan with cooking spray. Heat to medium-high heat. Pour ¼ cup batter for each pancake and cook for approximately 2 to 3 minutes. When bubbles appear on the upper surface, flip the pancakes. Continue cooking until the second side is golden brown, about 2 minutes.

As you make more pancakes, keep the finished pancakes in the warmed oven on a cookie sheet, separated with parchment paper. When ready to serve, add a few drops of fresh lemon juice over the pancakes, if desired.

Nutrition information per serving ($^1/_5$ of recipe): calories: 260, total fat: 8g, saturated fat: 1g, protein: 9g, carbohydrates: 39g, dietary fiber: 3g

BREAKFAST

berry surprise pancakes

(Courtesy of American Institute for Cancer Research, www.aicr.org)

Serves 6 (24 small pancakes)

1 cup unbleached all-purpose flour
⅔ cup whole-wheat pastry flour
1 teaspoon baking soda
¼ teaspoon salt
2 cups buttermilk
1 large egg
1 large egg white
8 ounces fresh blueberries
1 small container fresh raspberries (about 1 cup)
1 pound strawberries, hulled and chopped
Sugar (preferably superfine), to taste
Canola oil spray, as needed

➤ In a mixing bowl, whisk together the all-purpose and whole-wheat flours, baking soda, and salt. In a small bowl, whisk together the buttermilk, egg, and egg white until blended. Pour liquid ingredients into dry ones, whisking just until blended. (Do not over-mix, some small lumps are fine.) Stir in the blueberries. Set batter aside.

In a blender or food processor, puree raspberries and strawberries until smooth. Taste and, if too tart, gradually add sugar (½ teaspoon at a time) until lightly sweetened. Transfer to a serving bowl and set aside.

Spray a large griddle or frying pan with canola oil spray. Heat over medium-high heat. Using a ¼ measuring cup, pour batter into pan, making 4-inch pancakes. Cook until tiny bubbles appear on the top of each pancake and the bottom is lightly browned, 3 to 4 minutes. Turn and cook until pancake resists when pressed lightly in the center and bottoms are lightly browned. Serve immediately with the pureed berries for a topping.

. . . .

Nutrition information per serving (4 small pancakes): calories: 245, total fat: 4g, saturated fat: 1 g, protein: 10g, carbohydrates: 44g, dietary fiber: 6g

BREAKFAST

banana oatmeal muffins

(Courtesy of American Institute for Cancer Research, www.aicr.org)

Serves 12

1 cup old-fashioned oats (not quick-cooking)

1 cup 1% or fat-free buttermilk

1½ cups whole-wheat pastry flour

1 teaspoon ground cinnamon

1 teaspoon baking powder

½ teaspoon baking soda

¼ teaspoon salt

1 large egg

½ cup applesauce

1 cup mashed ripe banana (2 or 3 bananas)

½ cup lightly packed light brown sugar

½ cup chopped walnuts

Canola oil spray, as needed

➤ In large mixing bowl, combine oats and buttermilk and set aside for 1 hour.

Preheat oven to 400°F. Drop foil liners into a 12-cavity muffin tin with 3-inch cups. Coat inside of liners generously with cooking spray and set aside. As an alternative, you can spray the muffin tin without using liners; this produces muffins with a chewier crust.

In small bowl, whisk together flour, cinnamon, baking powder, baking soda. and salt. Break egg into bowl with soaked oats and beat it lightly with fork, then mix it in. Add applesauce, banana, and sugar, then whisk until wet ingredients are well blended. Add dry ingredients, whisking just until they are combined: over-mixing makes muffins tough.

Spoon batter into prepared muffin tin. Sprinkle walnuts over tops of muffins. Bake for 20 minutes, or until bamboo skewer inserted into center of muffin comes out clean. Let sit for 3 minutes, then turn the muffins out onto wire rack and cool for 15 minutes. Serve warm.

Note: If not using liners, run a thin knife along the edges of the muffins before turning them out.

Nutrition information per serving (1 muffin): calories: 180, total fat: 4.5 g, saturated fat: 0.5 g, protein: 5g, carbohydrates: 30 g, dietary fiber: 4 g

BREAKFAST

strawberry-blueberry muffins

(Courtesy of American Institute for Cancer Research, www.aicr.org

Serves 12

3 tablespoons canola oil

⅓ cup unsweetened applesauce

½ cup sugar

2 eggs

1 teaspoon vanilla extract

1 cup fresh blueberries

1 cup chopped fresh strawberries

1 cup whole-wheat flour

1 cup unbleached all-purpose flour

2 teaspoons baking powder

¼ teaspoon salt

½ cup fat-free milk

Canola oil spray, as needed

➤ Preheat oven to 375°F. Spray 12-cup muffin tin with canola oil and set aside. In medium bowl, whisk together oil, applesauce, sugar, and eggs. Add vanilla, blueberries, and strawberries. In separate bowl, blend together flours, baking powder, and salt. Fold in half of the flour mixture, then half of the milk. Add remaining flour and milk, folding in just until blended. Scoop batter into prepared tins. Bake for 25 to 30 minutes, or until golden brown and inserted toothpick comes out dry. Allow muffins to cool for 20 minutes before removing from pan.

Nutrition information per serving (1 muffin): calories: 165, total fat: 5g, saturated fat: <1g, protein: 4g, carbohydrates: 28g, dietary fiber: 2g

red and yellow pepper omelets

Serves 2

1 teaspoon olive oil
1 sweet red pepper, thinly sliced
1 yellow pepper, thinly sliced
4 egg whites
½ teaspoon dried basil
¼ teaspoon black pepper
2 teaspoons grated Parmesan cheese, divided

➤ In a large non-stick frying pan over medium heat, warm oil; add the red peppers and yellow peppers; cook, stirring frequently for 4 to 5 minutes. Keep warm over low heat. In a small bowl, lightly whisk together the egg whites, basil, and black pepper. Coat a small non-stick frying pan with non-stick spray. Warm over medium-high heat for 1 minute. Add half of the egg mixture, swirling the pan to evenly coat the bottom. Cook for 30 seconds or until the eggs are set. Carefully loosen and flip; cook for 1 minute, or until firm. Sprinkle half of the peppers over the eggs. Fold to enclose the filling. Transfer to a plate. Sprinkle with 1 teaspoon of the Parmesan cheese. Repeat with the remaining egg mixture, peppers, and 1 teaspoon of Parmesan cheese.

Nutrition information per serving (1 omelet): calories: 90, total fat: 3g, saturated fat: 1g, protein: 9g, carbohydrates: 8g, dietary fiber: 2g

BREAKFAST

BREAKFAST

broccoli frittata

Serves 4

½ cup fat-free cottage cheese
2 cups fat-free egg substitute
1 large onion, diced
1 teaspoon olive oil
½ teaspoon dried dill
2 cups frozen chopped broccoli
2 teaspoon margarine, divided

➤ Mix cottage cheese and egg substitute together; set aside. In large non-stick frying pan over medium heat, sauté onions in oil for 5 minutes, or until soft. Add dill and broccoli; sauté for 5 minutes, or until broccoli mixture softens. Set vegetables aside. Wipe out frying pan. Add 1 teaspoon of margarine and swirl the pan to distribute it. Add half of the vegetable mixture, and then add half of the egg mixture; lift and rotate pan so that eggs are evenly distributed. As eggs set around the edges, lift them to allow uncooked portions to flow underneath. Turn heat to low, cover the pan, and cook until top is set. Invert onto a serving plate and cut into wedges. Repeat with remaining 1 teaspoon of margarine, vegetable mixture, and egg mixture.

Nutrition information per serving (1 frittata): calories: 150, total fat: 3g, saturated fat: 0g, protein: 19g, carbohydrates: 12g, dietary fiber: 3g

breakfast banana smoothie

(Courtesy of American Institute for Cancer Research, www.aicr.org)

Serves 2

2 medium bananas, peeled and sliced
1 (8 oz.) container fat-free plain yogurt
1½ cups skim milk
1 teaspoon toasted wheat germ
Dash of cinnamon or nutmeg

➤ In blender, combine bananas, yogurt, milk, and wheat germ. Blend until smooth. Pour mixture into chilled glasses. Sprinkle with cinnamon or nutmeg. Serve immediately.

Nutrition information per serving (½ of recipe): calories: 227, total fat: 1g, saturated fat: <1g, protein: 13g, carbohydrates: 47g, dietary fiber: 3g

BREAKFAST

BREAKFAST

black- and blueberry smoothie

Serves 4

2 cups blackberries
2 cups blueberries
1 cup fat-free plain yogurt
1 cup fat-free milk
1 teaspoon vanilla extract
2 cups ice

➤ Place all ingredients into blender and blend until smooth. Serve immediately.

Nutrition information per serving (¼ of recipe): calories: 120, total fat: 1g, saturated fat: 0g, protein: 6g, carbohydrates: 26g, dietary fiber: 5g

golden apple oatmeal

Serves 1

1 Golden Delicious apple, diced
⅓ cup apple juice
⅓ cup water
Dash of cinnamon
Dash of nutmeg
⅓ cup quick-cook rolled oats, uncooked

➤ Combine apples, juice, water, and seasonings; bring to a boil. Stir in rolled oats; cook for 1 minute. Cover and let stand for several minutes before serving.

Nutrition information per serving (1 bowl): calories: 200, total fat: 2g, saturated fat: 0g, protein: 4g, carbohydrates: 45g, dietary fiber: 6g

maple raisin granola

(Courtesy of American Institute for Cancer Research, www.aicr.org)

Serves 10

3 cups old-fashioned rolled oats
¼ cup whole-wheat flour
½ teaspoon cinnamon
Pinch of salt
½ cup pure maple syrup
⅓ cup canola oil
1 teaspoon vanilla extract
1 cup raisins
Canola oil spray, as needed

➤ Preheat oven to 300°F. Lightly coat baking sheet with canola oil spray. In large bowl, combine oats, flour, cinnamon, and salt. In separate bowl, whisk together syrup, oil, and vanilla extract. Add to oat mixture, stirring well to coat. Spread mixture across baking sheet. Bake for 30 minutes.

Remove tray from oven. Sprinkle granola with raisins. Using a large spoon or spatula, mix raisins and granola, breaking up any lumps. Return to oven and continue baking for an additional 20 minutes. Allow granola to cool completely. Store in airtight container in refrigerator.

Nutrition information per serving (1/10 of recipe): calories: 259, total fat: 9g, saturated fat: <1g, protein: 5g, carbohydrates: 42g, dietary fiber: 4g

modified macaroni 'n cheese

(Courtesy of American Institute for Cancer Research, www.aicr.org)

Serves 8

2 cups uncooked whole-wheat elbow macaroni
1 tablespoon butter or margarine
1 onion, finely chopped
1 garlic clove, minced
1 small red bell pepper, finely sliced
1 small green bell pepper, finely sliced
1½ cups low-fat milk
¼ cup grated Parmesan cheese
1 cup shredded reduced-fat sharp or extra-sharp cheddar cheese
½ cup fat-free sour cream
½ teaspoon paprika
Salt and freshly ground black pepper, to taste

➤ In large saucepan, cook macaroni according to package directions. Drain and return to pan. Set aside. In large skillet, heat butter or margarine over medium heat; sauté onion and garlic until onion is translucent. Add bell peppers and sauté for 2 more minutes, stirring constantly. Add to macaroni. In small bowl, combine milk, Parmesan, cheddar, and sour cream. Add to macaroni and cook for 10 minutes over low or medium heat, stirring constantly, until cheese is completely melted and macaroni is piping hot. Add salt and pepper to taste. Sprinkle with paprika to garnish.

Nutrition information per serving (⅛ of recipe): calories: 198, total fat: 6g, saturated fat: 4g, protein: 11g, carbohydrates: 27g, dietary fiber: 3g

LUNCH

apple tuna sandwich

(Fruits & Veggies—More Matters® recipes appear courtesy of Produce for Better Health Foundation (PBH). This recipe meets Centers for Disease Control & Prevention's (CDC) strict nutrition guidelines as a healthy recipe. Find this recipe and others like it online at www.FruitAandVeggiesMoreMatters.org.)

Serves 3

2 (6 oz.) cans unsalted tuna in water, drained

1 medium apple, chopped

1 celery stalk, peeled and chopped

¼ cup low-fat vanilla yogurt

1 teaspoon prepared mustard

1 teaspoon honey

6 slices whole-wheat bread

6 lettuce leaves

6 slices tomato

➤ Combine and mix the tuna, apple, celery, yogurt, mustard, and honey. Spread ½ cup of the mixture on each of three bread slices. Top each slice of bread with lettuce, tomato, and remaining bread. Cut sandwiches in half or as desired.

Nutrition information per serving (1 sandwich): calories: 330, total fat: 4g, saturated fat: 1g, protein: 38g, carbohydrates: 37g, dietary fiber: 6g

red, white, and green grilled cheese

(Courtesy of the National Heart, Lung, and Blood Institute (NHLBI), www.nhlbi.nih.gov)

Serves 4

1 teaspoon garlic, minced (about ½ clove)

1 small onion, minced (about ½ cup)

2 cups frozen cut spinach, thawed and drained
   or 2 (10 oz.) bags fresh leaf spinach, rinsed

¼ teaspoon ground black pepper

8 slices whole-wheat bread

1 medium tomato, rinsed, cut into 4 slices

1 cup shredded part-skim mozzarella cheese

Canola oil spray, as needed

➤ Preheat oven to 400°F. Place a large baking sheet in the oven to preheat for about 10 minutes. Heat garlic with cooking spray in a medium sauté pan over medium heat. Cook until soft, but not browned. Add onions, and continue to cook until the onions are soft, but not browned. Add spinach, and toss gently. Cook until the spinach is heated throughout. Season with pepper and set aside to cool.

When the spinach and onions are cool, assemble each sandwich with one slice of bread on the bottom, one tomato slice, ½ cup of spinach mixture, ¼ cup of cheese, and a second slice of bread on the top. Spray the preheated nonstick baking sheet with cooking spray. Place the sandwiches on the baking sheet. Bake for 10 minutes, or until the bottom of each sandwich is browned. Carefully flip sandwiches and bake for an additional 5 minutes, or until both sides are browned. Serve immediately.

Note: For picky eaters, start with less spinach in the sandwich and work your way up.

....

Nutrition information per serving (1 sandwich): calories: 254, total fat: 8g, saturated fat: 4g, protein: 17g, carbohydrates: 29g, dietary fiber: 6g

turkey-apple gyros

Serves 6

1 medium Golden Delicious apple, cored and thinly sliced

2 tablespoons fresh lemon juice

1 cup thinly sliced onion

1 medium red bell pepper, cut into thin strips

1 medium green bell pepper, cut into thin strips

1 teaspoon olive oil

8 ounces cooked turkey breast, cut into thin strips

1 garlic clove, minced

½ cup plain low-fat yogurt

6 whole-wheat pita bread rounds, lightly toasted

➤ Toss apple with lemon juice; set aside. In a large nonstick skillet, sauté onion and peppers in hot oil, stirring frequently until crisp-tender. Add turkey to skillet and stir until heated through. Stir in apple mixture. Add garlic to yogurt and mix. Fold pitas in half and fill with turkey mixture. Drizzle with yogurt mixture.

Nutrition information per serving (1 sandwich): calories: 260, total fat: 4g, saturated fat: 1g, protein: 24g, carbohydrates: 36g, dietary fiber: 5g

pita pizza

(Courtesy of the National Heart, Lung, and Blood Institute (NHLBI), www.nhlbi.nih.gov)

Serves 4

4 (6½-inch) whole-wheat pitas
1 cup Super Quick Chunky Tomato Sauce (page 102)
1 cup grilled boneless, skinless chicken breast, diced (about
    2 small breasts)
1 cup broccoli, rinsed, chopped, and cooked
2 tablespoons grated Parmesan cheese
1 tablespoon fresh basil, rinsed, dried, and chopped
    (or 1 teaspoon dried)

➤ Preheat oven or toaster oven to 450°F. For each pizza, spread ¼ cup tomato sauce on a pita and top with ¼ cup chicken, ¼ cup broccoli, ½ tablespoon Parmesan cheese, and ¼ tablespoon chopped basil. Place pitas on a nonstick baking sheet and bake for about 5 to 8 minutes until golden brown and chicken is heated through. Serve immediately.

Nutrition information per serving (1 pita pizza): calories: 275, total fat: 5g, saturated fat: 1g, protein: 20g, carbohydrates: 41g, dietary fiber: 7g

tuscan chickpea soup

(Courtesy of American Institute for Cancer Research, www.aicr.org)

Serves 6

2 (15 oz.) cans chickpeas, rinsed and drained

2 large whole garlic cloves, peeled

1 (14¼ oz.) can reduced-sodium vegetable broth

2 cups water

2 teaspoons extra-virgin olive oil

1 medium onion, chopped

2 tablespoons tomato paste

1 teaspoon chopped fresh rosemary

2 teaspoons extra-virgin olive oil, for garnish (optional)

1 teaspoon lemon juice, for garnish (optional)

2½ tablespoons minced flat-leaf parsley, for garnish (optional)

Salt and freshly ground black pepper, to taste

➤ Place chickpeas and garlic in a large saucepan. Pour broth and 2 cups cold water into a pot and bring to a boil over medium-high heat. Reduce heat and simmer, covered, until beans are very soft, about 20 minutes. Let the soup sit for 10 minutes to cool slightly.

Meanwhile, heat oil in a small skillet over medium-high heat. Add onion and cook, stirring often, until onion is soft, about 5 minutes. Transfer mixture to blender. Add chickpeas, garlic, liquid, tomato paste, and rosemary. Puree until smooth (this may need to be done in two batches). Make soup smooth or leave some texture, whichever you prefer. Season to taste with salt and pepper.

To serve, ladle soup into bowls. Garnish each either by drizzling ½ teaspoon of olive oil over the soup or by mixing in 1 teaspoon lemon juice. Sprinkle with parsley.

Nutrition information per serving (1 cup): calories: 142, total fat: 3g, saturated fat: <1g, protein: 8g, carbohydrates: 21g, dietary fiber: 5g

old-fashioned tomato soup

(Courtesy of American Institute for Cancer Research, www.aicr.org)

Serves 4

1 tablespoon butter
1 onion, finely chopped
2 large garlic cloves, chopped
1 (28 oz.) can diced tomatoes
1 tablespoon sugar
1 teaspoon dried thyme
⅛ teaspoon ground mace
Pinch of cayenne pepper
½ cup fat-free half-and-half cream
3 tablespoons snipped dill, for garnish (optional)
Salt and freshly ground black pepper, to taste

➤ Melt the butter in a small Dutch oven over medium-high heat. Sauté the onion until translucent, about 4 minutes. Add the garlic and sauté until the onions are golden, 5 to 6 minutes. Add the tomatoes (with their juices), sugar, thyme, mace, and cayenne. Bring to a boil, cover, and simmer the soup until the tomatoes and onion are soft, about 15 minutes.

Let the soup sit for 20 minutes, uncovered. Transfer it to a blender and reduce the mixture to a puree, either pulpy or completely smooth, as desired. Blend in the half-and-half. Season the soup to taste with salt and pepper.

Serve the soup hot, sprinkling one-fourth of the dill over each bowl, if desired.

Nutrition information per serving (1 bowl): calories: 339, total fat: 1g, saturated fat: 3g, protein: 3g, carbohydrate: 18g, dietary fiber: <1g

LUNCH

beef barley and lima bean soup

Serves 6

1 cup chopped onion

1 cup chopped carrots

1 (14½ oz.) can low-sodium beef broth

1 pound lean beef stew meat, cut in ½-inch cubes

4 cups water

¼ cup dry pearl barley

½ teaspoon salt

¼ teaspoon pepper

3 cups cooked (1 cup dry) large lima beans

   or 2 (15 oz.) cans butter beans, drained

2 tablespoons minced parsley

➤ Place onion and carrots in a large dry saucepan. Cook over high heat, stirring frequently until vegetables start to brown and stick. Add ½ cup broth; stir to release brown bits. Cook until liquid evaporates and vegetables begin to stick again, about 5 minutes. Add ½ cup broth and continue cooking until liquid evaporates and vegetables are soft and golden brown. Add meat and cook until no longer pink. Stir in remaining broth, water, barley, salt, and pepper. Simmer, covered, for 25 minutes. Add beans and parsley; cook for 10 minutes or until barley is soft.

Nutrition information per serving (¹/₆ of recipe): calories: 280, total fat: 6g, saturated fat: 2g, protein: 24g, carbohydrate: 31 g, dietary fiber: 9g

confetti appleslaw

Serves 8

2 tablespoons orange concentrate, defrosted

1 red apple, unpeeled, cored, and diced

4 cups shredded cabbage

2 small red onions, finely shredded

1 red or green sweet pepper, thinly sliced

3 tablespoons raisins

1 tablespoon reduced-calorie mayonnaise

½ cup plain low-fat yogurt

½ teaspoon dry mustard

⅛ teaspoon paprika

⅛ teaspoon freshly ground black pepper

➤ In a large bowl, stir together juice concentrate and diced apple. Add cabbage, onion, pepper, and raisins. In a small bowl, stir together mayonnaise, yogurt, mustard, paprika, and pepper. Add to vegetable mixture. Cover tightly and refrigerate until ready to serve.

Nutrition information per serving (⅛ of recipe): calories: 60, total fat: 5g, saturated fat: 0g, protein: 2g, carbohydrate: 13 g, dietary fiber: 2g

outtasight salad

(Courtesy of ChooseMyPlate.gov)

Serves 4

Dressing:
¼ cup fat-free plain yogurt
1 tablespoon orange juice
1½ teaspoons white vinegar

Salad:
2 cups salad greens of your choice
1 cup chopped vegetables (such as tomatoes, cucumbers, carrots, and green beans)
1 cup juice-packed pineapple chunks, drained or fresh orange segments
2 tablespoons raisins or dried cranberries
2 tablespoons chopped nuts of your choice

➤ *Dressing:*
In a small bowl, mix all ingredients. Refrigerate until ready to serve.

➤ *Salad:*
Put mixed salad greens on a large platter or in a salad bowl. In a large bowl, mix chopped vegetables and pineapple or orange segments. Add dressing and stir. Spoon mixture over salad greens. Top with raisins and nuts.

Nutrition information per serving (1 cup): calories: 100, total fat: 2.5g, saturated fat: 0g, protein: 2g

chicken quesadillas with red and green salsa

(Courtesy of the National Heart, Lung, and Blood Institute (NHLBI), www.nhlbi.nih.gov)

Serves 4

Salsa:

4 medium tomatoes, rinsed and diced (about 2 cups)

½ cup red onion, diced

1 medium jalapeño chili pepper, rinse and split lengthwise, remove seeds and white membrane, and mince (about 2 tablespoons)

2 tablespoons lime juice (about 4 limes)

2 tablespoons fresh cilantro, rinsed, dried, and chopped (or 2 teaspoons dried coriander)

1 teaspoon ground cumin

Quesadillas:

12 ounces boneless, skinless chicken breast, cut into thin strips

4 (10-inch) whole-wheat tortillas

¼ teaspoon salt

½ teaspoon chili sauce

2 ounces pepper jack cheese, shredded (about ½ cup)

1 tablespoon pine nuts, toasted (optional)

Canola oil spray, as needed

➤ *Salsa:*

Combine all ingredients and toss well. Chill in refrigerator for at least 15 minutes. (Salsa can be made up to one day in advance and refrigerated.)

DINNER

➤ *Quesadillas:*

Preheat oven broiler on high temperature, with the rack 3 inches from heat source. Cut chicken into thin strips, and place them on a baking sheet coated with cooking spray. Broil for 8 to 10 minutes. To assemble the quesadillas, place four whole-wheat tortillas on the countertop or table. Top each with one-quarter of the sliced cooked chicken, salt, chili sauce, cheese, and pine nuts (optional). Fold tortillas in half to close and carefully transfer to a baking sheet lined with parchment or wax paper. Bake quesadillas at 350°F for 5 to 10 minutes or until the cheese is melted. Serve one quesadilla with ½ cup salsa on the side.

Note: For less spice, use green bell pepper in place of jalapeño pepper.

Nutrition information per serving (1 quesadilla and ½ cup salsa): calories: 339, total fat: 11g, saturated fat: 3g, protein: 26g, carbohydrates: 32g, dietary fiber: 4g

orzo skillet

(Fruits & Veggies—More Matters® recipes appear courtesy of Produce for Better Health Foundation (PBH). This recipe meets Centers for Disease Control & Prevention's (CDC) strict nutrition guidelines as a healthy recipe. Find this recipe and others like it online at www. FruitAandVeggiesMoreMatters.org.)

Serves 4

1 pound ground turkey

2 cups canned, crushed tomato

1 cup diced onion

½ cup orzo pasta, uncooked

1 cup water

1 cup chopped green bell pepper

1 tablespoon chopped fresh cilantro

½ teaspoon chili powder

⅛ teaspoon hot sauce

1 (16 oz.) can pinto beans, rinsed and drained

➤ Cook ground turkey in a large skillet over medium heat, stirring occasionally, until browned. Drain. Stir in remaining ingredients. Heat to boiling; reduce heat. Cover and simmer for 15 minutes, stirring frequently until pasta is tender.

Nutrition information per serving (¼ of recipe): calories: 330, total fat: 3g, saturated fat: 1g, protein: 38g, carbohydrates: 42g, dietary fiber: 8g

DINNER

bean and vegetable enchilada casserole

(Courtesy of American Institute for Cancer Research, www.aicr.org)

Serves 8

1 tablespoon canola oil
1 medium bell pepper, chopped
1 large onion, chopped
2 cloves garlic, minced
1 (14 oz.) can black beans, drained and rinsed
1 (14 oz.) can pinto beans, drained and rinsed
1 (16 oz.) package frozen corn, thawed
1 (28 oz.) can pureed or crushed tomatoes
1 tablespoon chili powder
½ teaspoon ground cumin
12 corn tortillas
1 cup grated reduced-fat Jack cheese
Dash of hot sauce, to taste
Salt and freshly ground pepper, to taste

➤ Preheat oven to 350°F. In large saucepan, heat oil over medium heat and sauté bell pepper, onion, and garlic for 5 minutes. Add beans, corn, tomatoes, a dash of hot sauce, and seasonings (including salt and pepper, if desired). Reduce heat to low and simmer for 15 minutes.

Assemble casserole in a 9- x 13-inch baking dish. Cover bottom with one-third of bean mixture. Layer six tortillas on top of beans. Repeat once more, and then end with bean mixture on top. Sprinkle cheese on top and bake until hot and bubbly, about 30 to 40 minutes.

Nutrition information per serving (⅛ of recipe): calories: 320, total fat: 7g, saturated fat: 2g, protein: 15g, carbohydrates: 53g, dietary fiber: 11g

super meatballs with spicy red sauce

(Courtesy of American Institute for Cancer Research, www.aicr.org)

Serves 4

1 tablespoon extra-virgin olive oil

1 small onion, finely chopped

2–3 finely chopped garlic cloves

1 (28 oz.) can no-salt-added crushed tomatoes

1 (28 oz.) can no-salt-added whole plum tomatoes in
   tomato sauce

2 tablespoons dried oregano

¼ teaspoon red pepper flakes, or to taste

1 pound 93–95% lean ground beef

10 ounces frozen chopped spinach, defrosted and squeezed dry

¼ cup Italian seasoned dry breadcrumbs

¼ cup chopped flat-leaf parsley

2 tablespoons grated Parmesan cheese

1 large egg, at room temperature

⅛ teaspoon ground black pepper

➤ Heat oil in large Dutch oven over medium-high heat. Add onion and cook for 3 minutes, stirring occasionally. Add garlic and cook until onions are translucent, about 3 minutes, stirring so garlic does not burn. Add crushed tomatoes. Add whole tomatoes: hold one at a time over pot and squeeze it in your fist, crushing tomato through your fingers, then add sauce remaining in can. Add oregano and red pepper flakes. Simmer sauce, uncovered, for 20 minutes, stirring occasionally.

   While sauce simmers, in mixing bowl, combine meat, spinach, breadcrumbs, parsley, cheese, egg, and pepper, mixing until well combined.

Divide mixture into eight parts and form each loosely into a meatball. (Divide mixture into 16 parts for smaller meatballs, if desired.)

Gently drop uncooked meatballs into sauce, cover, reduce heat to medium-low, and simmer until meatballs are cooked through, about 40 minutes.

If not serving immediately, cool meatballs and sauce together in a big bowl until room temperature, then cover and refrigerate for up to 3 days. Reheat, covered, in large pot over medium heat, stirring occasionally.

Serve meatballs in a bowl over spaghetti, topped with Spicy Red Sauce.

Nutrition information per serving (¼ of recipe): calories: 380, total fat: 13g, saturated fat: 4g, protein: 36g, carbohydrates: 36g, dietary fiber: 9g

smoky mustard-maple salmon

(Courtesy of ChooseMyPlate.gov)

Serves 4

3 tablespoons Dijon mustard

1 tablespoon pure maple syrup

¼ teaspoon smoked paprika or ground chipotle pepper

¼ teaspoon freshly ground pepper

⅛ teaspoon salt

4 (4 oz.) skinless, center-cut salmon fillets

Canola oil spray, as needed

➤ Preheat oven to 450°F. Line a baking sheet with foil and coat with cooking spray. Combine mustard, maple syrup, paprika (or chipotle), pepper, and salt in a small bowl. Place salmon fillets on the prepared baking sheet. Spread the mustard mixture evenly over the salmon. Roast until just cooked through, approximately 8 to 12 minutes.

Note: As an alternative, try replacing the strawberry preserves and strawberries with apricot preserves and sliced fresh or canned, well-drained peaches. Smoked paprika is made from smoke-dried, red peppers and adds earthy, smoky flavor. It can be used in many types of savory dishes. Look for different types of paprika at large supermarkets or online.

Nutrition information per serving (1 fillet): 148 calories, total fat: 4g, saturated fat: 1g, protein: 23g, carbohydrates: 3 g, dietary fiber: 0g

DINNER

garden turkey meatloaf

(**Courtesy of National Heart, Lung, and Blood Institute,
www.nhlbi.nih.gov**)

Serves 4

Meatloaf:
2 cups assorted vegetables, chopped (such as mushrooms,
    zucchini, red bell peppers, or spinach)
12 ounces 99% lean ground turkey
½ cup whole-wheat breadcrumbs (or regular breadcrumbs)
¼ cup fat-free evaporated milk
¼ teaspoon ground black pepper
2 tablespoons ketchup
1 tablespoon fresh chives, rinsed, dried, and chopped
    (or 1 teaspoon dried)
1 tablespoon fresh parsley, rinsed, dried, and chopped
    (or 1 teaspoon dried)
Canola oil spray, as needed

Glaze:
1 tablespoon ketchup
1 tablespoon honey
1 tablespoon Dijon mustard

➤ Preheat oven to 350°F. Steam or lightly sauté the assortment of
vegetables. Combine vegetables and the rest of the meatloaf ingredients

in a large bowl. Mix well. Spray a loaf pan with cooking spray, and spread meatloaf mixture evenly in the pan. Combine all ingredients for glaze. Brush glaze on top of the meatloaf. Bake meatloaf in the oven for 45 to 50 minutes (to a minimum internal temperature of 165°F). Let stand for 5 minutes before cutting into eight even slices.

Note: For picky eaters, try chopping vegetables in a food processer to make them smaller (and "hidden").

....

Nutrition information per serving (2 slices): calories: 180, total fat: 0g, saturated fat: 0g, protein: 25g, carbohydrates: 17g, dietary fiber: 2g

DINNER

sweet and sour pork

(Courtesy of ChooseMyPlate.gov)

Serves 4

1 tablespoon minced, fresh ginger

4 teaspoons reduced-sodium soy sauce, divided

2 teaspoons plus 1 tablespoon rice wine or dry sherry, divided

1½ teaspoons plus 2 teaspoons cornstarch, divided

¼ teaspoon salt

⅛ teaspoon ground white pepper

1 pound trimmed boneless pork shoulder or butt, cut into ¼-inch thick, bite-sized slices

1 teaspoon sesame oil

2 tablespoons pineapple juice

2 tablespoons distilled white vinegar

1 tablespoon ketchup

1½ teaspoons light brown sugar

2 tablespoons peanut or canola oil, divided

½ cup sliced carrot (¼-inch thick)

1 small tomato, thinly sliced into wedges

¼ cup finely chopped scallions

2 cups chopped fresh pineapple (bite-sized pieces) or drained canned pineapple chunks

➤ Combine ginger, 2 teaspoons of soy sauce, 2 teaspoons of rice wine (or sherry), 1½ teaspoons of cornstarch, salt, and pepper in a medium bowl.

Stir in pork and sesame oil until well combined. Combine pineapple juice, vinegar, ketchup, and brown sugar in a small bowl. Stir in the remaining soy sauce, rice wine (or sherry), and cornstarch.

Heat a 14-inch flat-bottomed wok over high heat until a bead of water vaporizes within 1 to 2 seconds of contact. Swirl 1 tablespoon peanut (or canola) oil into the wok. Carefully add the pork and spread in one layer. Cook undisturbed, letting the pork begin to sear, for 1½ minutes. Then, using a metal spatula, stir-fry until the pork is lightly browned but not cooked through, about 1 minute.

Transfer the pork to a plate. Swirl the remaining oil into the wok, add carrots and stir-fry for 30 seconds. Return the pork with any juices to the wok. Add tomato and scallions and stir-fry for 30 seconds. Swirl in the pineapple juice mixture, add pineapple, and stir-fry until the pork is just cooked through and the sauce is lightly thickened, approximately 1 to 2 minutes more.

Nutrition information per serving (1¼ cups): calories: 313, total fat: 17g, saturated fat: 5g, protein: 19g, carbohydrates: 21g, dietary fiber: 2g

DINNER

baked pork chops with apple cranberry sauce

(Courtesy of National Heart, Lung, and Blood Institute,
www.nhlbi.nih.gov)

Serves 4

Pork Chops:
4 boneless pork chops (about 3 ounces each)
¼ teaspoon ground black pepper
¼ teaspoon fresh orange zest (use a grater to take a thin layer of
    skin off the orange; save the orange for garnish)
½ tablespoon olive oil

Sauce:
¼ cup low-sodium chicken broth
1 medium apple, peeled and grated (about 1 cup, use a grater to
    make thin layers of apple)
½ cinnamon stick (or ⅛ teaspoon ground cinnamon)
1 bay leaf
½ cup dried cranberries (or raisins)
½ cup 100% orange juice

➤ Preheat oven to 350°F. Season pork chops with pepper and orange zest.
In a large sauté pan, heat olive oil over medium heat. Add pork chops,
and cook until browned on one side, about 2 minutes. Turn over and
brown the second side, an additional 2 minutes. Remove pork chops
from the pan, place them on a nonstick baking sheet, and put in the
oven to cook for an additional 10 minutes (to a minimum internal

temperature of 160°F). Add chicken broth to the sauté pan and stir to loosen the flavorful brown bits. Set aside.

Meanwhile, place grated apples, cinnamon stick, and bay leaf in a small saucepan. Cook over medium heat until the apples begin to soften. Add cranberries (or raisins), orange juice, and saved broth with flavorful brown bits. Bring to a boil, and then lower to a gentle simmer. Simmer for up to 10 minutes or until the cranberries are plump and the apples are tender. Remove the cinnamon stick. Peel the orange used for the zest, and cut it into eight sections for garnish.

Serve one pork chop with ¼ cup of sauce and two orange segments.

Note: If your children would prefer this dish without the sauce on top, serve a plain pork chop with separate sides of unsweetened applesauce, dried cranberries, and orange segments.

. . . .

Nutrition information per serving (1 pork chop, ¼ cup sauce, 2 orange segments): calories: 232, total fat: 7g, saturated fat: 2g, protein: 18g, carbohydrates: 25g, dietary fiber: 2g

DINNER

cornbread-crusted turkey

....

(Courtesy of National Heart, Lung, and Blood Institute,
www.nhlbi.nih.gov)

Serves 4

1 cup low-fat buttermilk
1 tablespoon Dijon mustard
4 skinless turkey fillets (3 ounces each)
1 cup cornbread crumbs
1 egg white (or liquid egg white)
1 cup low-sodium chicken broth
1 tablespoon cornstarch
1 pound frozen baby carrots
1 tablespoon fresh sage, rinsed, dried, and chopped
   (or 1 teaspoon dried)
1 tablespoon butter

➤ Preheat oven to 350°F. Combine buttermilk and Dijon mustard. Mix
well. Add turkey fillets to buttermilk mixture to marinate for 5 to
10 minutes while preparing cornbread. Grind cornbread in a food
processor, or use your fingers to make coarse crumbs. Place breadcrumbs
on a baking sheet, and dry in a 300°F oven or toaster oven for 4 to 5
minutes. Do not brown. Pour breadcrumbs into a dry, shallow dish. Put
egg white in a separate bowl. Remove turkey from the buttermilk, and
dip each fillet first in the egg white and then in the cornbread crumbs
to coat (be sure to discard leftover buttermilk mixture and cornbread
crumbs). Place breaded turkey fillets on a baking sheet, and bake for

10 to 15 minutes (to a minimum internal temperature of 165°F). While the turkey is cooking, combine chicken broth, cornstarch, carrots, sage, and butter in a medium saucepan. Bring to a boil over high heat, stirring occasionally. Lower temperature to a simmer. Simmer gently for about 5 minutes, or until the butter is melted, the sauce is thick, and the carrots are warm. Serve each 3-ounce turkey fillet with 1 cup of carrots and sauce mixture.

Serve with a baked or roasted sweet potato.

Nutrition information per serving (3 ounces of turkey, 1 cup carrots and sauce mixture): calories: 285, total fat: 6g, saturated fat: 3g, protein: 29g, carbohydrates: 29g, dietary fiber: 3g

DINNER

super quick chunky tomato sauce

(Courtesy of the National Heart, Lung, and Blood Institute (NHLBI),
www.nhlbi.nih.gov)

Serves 12

2 teaspoons olive oil

1 teaspoon garlic, chopped (about 1 clove)

1 (12 oz.) jar roasted red peppers, drained and diced
(or fresh roasted red peppers)

2 (14½ oz.) cans no-salt-added diced tomatoes

1 (5½ oz.) can low-sodium tomato juice

1 tablespoon fresh basil, rinsed, dried, and chopped
(or 1 teaspoon dried)

¼ teaspoon ground black pepper

➤ In a medium saucepan, heat olive oil and garlic over medium heat.
Cook until soft, but not browned, about 30 seconds. Add diced red
peppers and continue to cook for 2 to 3 minutes, until the peppers
begin to sizzle. Add tomatoes, tomato juice, basil, and pepper. Bring
to a boil. Simmer for 10 minutes, or until the sauce thickens slightly.
(Sauce can be pureed for picky eaters.) Use immediately, or refrigerate
in a tightly sealed container for 3 to 5 days or freeze for 1 to 2 months.

Nutrition information per serving (½ cup): calories: 31, total fat: 1g, saturated fat: 0g, protein: 1g, carbohydrates: 4g, dietary fiber: 1g

spiced toasted almonds

(Courtesy of American Institute for Cancer Research, www.aicr.org)

Serves 8 (makes 2 cups)

1 tablespoon dried thyme leaves

1 teaspoon kosher or sea salt

¼ teaspoon red (cayenne) pepper, or to taste

2 teaspoons canola oil

2 cups whole, unblanched almonds

Canola oil spray, as needed

➤ Preheat oven to 400°F. In large, shallow bowl, combine thyme, salt, pepper, and oil. Set aside.

Place nuts in medium bowl. While tossing with fork, lightly spray with canola oil so all surfaces are coated. Lightly coat baking sheet with canola oil spray. Turn nuts onto sheet and spread evenly across surface. Place baking sheet in center of the oven. Toast until nuts are lightly browned and fragrant, about 8 minutes. Occasionally shake pan to shift nuts and prevent scorching (be careful not to let nuts get too dark or they'll taste burned). Remove from oven and immediately add hot nuts to spice mixture. Stir for a few minutes to coat the nuts thoroughly. Taste and adjust the seasonings. Serve warm or at room temperature. Nuts can be sealed and stored for up to two weeks. Reheat in a hot oven.

Nutritional information per serving (¼ cup): calories: 223, total fat: 19g, saturated fat: 1g, protein: 7g, carbohydrates: 7g, dietary fiber: 4g

SNACKS

toasted whole-wheat pita wedges

(Courtesy of American Institute for Cancer Research, www.aicr.org)

Serves 4

2 whole-wheat pita breads (6 inches)
2 tablespoons Parmesan cheese
Olive oil spray, as needed

➤ Preheat oven to 350°F. Separate halves of each pita bread, then cut each half into eight wedges.

On large baking sheet, place wedges in a single layer. Spray lightly with olive oil. Sprinkle with Parmesan cheese. Bake for 15 minutes.

Nutritional information per serving (¼ of recipe): calories: 97, total fat: 2g, saturated fat: <1g, protein: 4g, carbohydrates: 18 g, dietary fiber: 2g

fresh salsa

(Courtesy of National Heart, Lung, and Blood Institute, www.nhlbi.nih.gov)

Serves 8

6 tomatoes, preferably Roma (or 3 large tomatoes)
½ medium onion, finely chopped
1 clove garlic, finely minced
2 serrano or jalapeño peppers, finely chopped
Juice of 1 lime
⅛ teaspoon oregano, finely crushed
⅛ teaspoon salt
⅛ teaspoon pepper
½ avocado, diced (black skin)

➤ Combine all ingredients in a bowl and toss well. Serve immediately or refrigerate and serve within 4 to 5 hours.

Nutrition information per serving (½ cup): calories: 42, total fat: 2g, saturated fat: less than 1g

SNACKS

cucumber yogurt dip

Serves 6

    2 large cucumbers
    2 cups plain low-fat yogurt
    ½ cup fat-free sour cream
    1 tablespoon lemon juice
    1 tablespoon fresh dill
    1 garlic clove, chopped
    1 cup cherry tomatoes
    1 cup broccoli florets
    1 cup baby carrots

➤ Peel, seed, and grate one cucumber. Slice other cucumber and set aside. Mix yogurt, grated cucumber, sour cream, lemon juice, dill, and garlic in a serving bowl. Chill for 1 hour. Arrange tomatoes, cucumbers, broccoli, and carrots on a colorful platter. Serve with cucumber dip.

Nutrition information per serving (¹⁄₆ of recipe): calories: 100, total fat: 2g, saturated fat: 1g, protein: 7g, carbohydrates: 17g, dietary fiber: 2g

chickpea dip

Serves 4

3 cloves garlic

¼ cup plain low-fat yogurt

1 tablespoon fresh lemon juice

1 teaspoon olive oil

¼ teaspoon salt

¼ teaspoon paprika

⅛ teaspoon pepper

1 (19 oz.) can chickpeas, drained

➤ Put all ingredients into a food processor and blend until smooth. Serve at room temperature with pita chips, crackers, carrots, or other dipping vegetables.

Nutrition information per serving (¼ of recipe): calories: 140, total fat: 4g, saturated fat: 0g, protein: 7g, carbohydrates: 21g, dietary fiber: 5g

ranch hand nachos

Serves 5

1 pound small red bliss potatoes, skins on
8 ounces extra-lean ground turkey breast
½ teaspoon chili powder
⅔ cup reduced-fat cheddar cheese, shredded
1 cup iceberg lettuce, shredded
1 medium tomato, diced
¾ cup cucumber, peeled and diced
1 tablespoon cilantro, chopped
¾ cup salsa, mild
Canola oil spray, as needed

➤ Slice potatoes into small circles. Coat them with cooking oil spray for 3 seconds. Bake in the oven at 450°F for 25 to 30 minutes, depending on desired darkness. Brown ground turkey breast with chili powder in pan over medium heat for 8 to 10 minutes. Remove potatoes from the oven and turn off. Place the potatoes on a small oven-safe platter or long dish. Top with cheese and turkey, then put back in the oven to melt, about 2 minutes. Remove from oven and top with lettuce, tomato, cucumber, cilantro, and salsa.

Nutrition information per serving (¹/₅ of recipe): calories: 178, total fat: 2.8g, saturated fat: 0.7g, protein: 18g, carbohydrates: 22g, dietary fiber: 4g

papaya boats

Serves 4

2 ripe papayas
1 cup Mandarin oranges, drained
1 banana (small and ripe), sliced
1 kiwi, peeled and sliced
½ cup blueberries
½ cup strawberries
¾ cup fat-free vanilla yogurt
2 teaspoons chopped fresh mint

➤ Cut papayas in half lengthwise; scoop out seeds. Place oranges, banana, kiwi, and berries in each papaya half. Combine yogurt and mint; mix well and spoon over fruit before serving. Garnish with mint sprigs, if desired.

Nutrition information per serving (1 boat): calories: 170, total fat: 1g, saturated fat: 0g, protein: 4g, carbohydrates: 40g, dietary fiber: 5g

SNACKS

apricot bar cookies

(Courtesy of American Institute for Cancer Research, www.aicr.org)

Serves 16

1 cup quick-cooking rolled oats

1 cup whole-wheat flour

⅓ cup packed brown sugar

½ teaspoon cinnamon

¼ teaspoon salt

¼ teaspoon baking soda

⅓ cup canola oil

5 tablespoons apple juice, divided

½ cup apricot jam, preferably fruit-sweetened

1 (7 oz.) package dried apricots, diced

Canola oil spray, as needed

➤ Preheat oven to 350°F. Spray 9- x 9-inch baking pan with cooking spray. In large bowl, mix together oats, flour, sugar, cinnamon, salt, and baking soda until well combined. In small bowl, whisk together oil and 3 tablespoons juice and pour over oat mixture, blending well until moist and crumbly. Reserve ¾ cup for topping. Press the remainder evenly into prepared pan. In small bowl, blend jam with remaining 2 tablespoons apple juice. Stir in dried apricots. Spread evenly over crust. Sprinkle reserved crumb mixture over apricots, lightly pressing down with fingers. Bake for 35 minutes or until golden. Cool in pan on wire rack. Cut into bars.

Nutrition information per serving (1 bar): calories: 162, total fat: 5g, saturated fat: <1g, protein: 2g, carbohydrates: 28g, dietary fiber: 2g

whole-wheat date walnut bars

(Courtesy of American Institute for Cancer Research, www.aicr.org)

Serves 16

¾ cup whole-wheat flour

¼ teaspoon baking powder

¼ teaspoon baking soda

⅛ teaspoon salt

1 large egg

¼ cup honey

2 tablespoons canola oil

½ teaspoon grated orange peel

3 tablespoons applesauce

⅔ cup pitted and chopped dates

⅓ cup chopped walnuts

Canola oil spray, as needed

➤ Preheat oven to 350°F. Lightly spray 8-inch baking pan with canola oil spray and set aside. In large bowl, mix flour, baking powder, baking soda, and salt. In small bowl, mix egg, honey, canola oil, orange peel, and applesauce. Stir egg mixture into dry ingredients until blended. Stir in dates and walnuts. Spread mixture into prepared pan. Bake until a clean dry knife inserted into center comes out clean, about 25 minutes. Cool in pan on wire rack. Cut into 16 squares.

Nutrition information per serving (1 bar): calories: 91, total fat: 4g, saturated fat: <1g, protein: 2g, carbohydrates: 14g, dietary fiber: 1g

black bean brownies

(Courtesy of American Institute for Cancer Research, www.aicr.org)

Serves 16

1 (15 oz.) can reduced-sodium black beans, rinsed and drained

3 large eggs

3 tablespoons canola oil

¼ cup unsweetened cocoa powder

Pinch of salt

½ tablespoon vanilla extract

⅔ cup light brown sugar, packed

3 tablespoons bittersweet or dark chocolate chips

Canola oil spray, as needed

➤ Preheat oven to 350°F. Coat 8-inch baking pan with canola oil spray. In a food processor, place beans, eggs, canola oil, cocoa powder, salt, vanilla, and brown sugar and blend until smooth. Remove blade and carefully stir in chocolate chips. Transfer mixture to prepared pan. Bake for 30 to 35 minutes, or until a clean dry knife inserted in center comes out clean. Cool before cutting into squares.

Nutrition information per serving (1 brownie): calories: 110, total fat: 5g, saturated fat: 1g, protein: 3g, carbohydrates: 15g, dietary fiber: 2g

frozen fruit cups

(Courtesy of ChooseMyPlate.gov)

Makes 18 fruit cups

3 bananas, mashed

24 ounces fat-free strawberry (or plain) yogurt

10 ounces frozen strawberries, thawed, undrained

1 (8 oz.) can crushed pineapple, undrained

➤ Line muffin tins with paper baking cups (18 total). In a large mixing bowl, add mashed bananas, yogurt, strawberries, and pineapple. Spoon the mixture into the muffin tin and freeze for at least 3 hours, or until firm.

Remove the frozen cups and store them in a plastic bag in the freezer. Before serving, remove paper cups.

KID CREATIONS

KID CREATIONS

frozen bananas

(Courtesy of ChooseMyPlate.gov)

Serves 1

1 banana
1 wooden popsicle stick for each banana
Plastic wrap

➤ Peel and cut bananas in half. Put a wooden stick into each banana. Wrap in plastic wrap and freeze. Once frozen, peel off the plastic and enjoy.

KID CREATIONS

frozen graham cracker sandwiches

(Courtesy of ChooseMyPlate.gov)

Serves 5–6

> 2 bananas
> 1 cup peanut butter
> 10–12 graham crackers
> Plastic wrap

➤ Mash the bananas with a fork or potato masher. Add the peanut butter to the mashed bananas and mix well. Spread the mixture on a graham cracker and cover it with a second cracker. Wrap each graham cracker sandwich with a piece of plastic wrap and freeze. Once frozen, simply peel off the plastic and enjoy.

yogurt parfait

Makes 1–2 parfaits

> 1 banana
> 2 cups low-fat plain yogurt
> 1 cup berries (such as raspberries or blueberries)
> ½ cup Maple Raisin Granola (page 74)

➤ Mash up the banana with a fork and blend it in with the yogurt. Alternate layers of the yogurt-banana mixture and berries into tall, clear glasses. Sprinkle the granola on top of the yogurt parfait.

trail mix

Makes 8 cups

2 cups unsweetened whole-grain dry oat cereal or air-popped popcorn
¼ cup chopped dates
¼ cup golden raisins
½ cup dried cranberries
½ cup yogurt raisins
2 cups banana chips
1½ cups mixed nuts

➤ In a large bowl, combine the oat cereal (or popcorn) and chopped dates. Mix them together and then add the golden raisins, dried cranberries, and yogurt raisins. Again, stir the trail mix. Add the banana chips and mixed nuts to the mixture. Give the trail mix one final toss using your clean hands. Scoop ½ cup servings in small storage bags and store them at room temperature for easy access. This makes it easy to grab a bag on the go or to toss in a lunch box.

Note: This recipe can tailored to meet your tastes by leaving out ingredients or replacing them with your favorite types of nuts, seeds, or dried fruit.

fruit and cheese kabobs

Assorted fruit pieces (such as grapes, watermelon, strawberries,
 cantaloupe, pineapple, or honeydew melon)
Cheddar cheese, cubed

➤ Cut any larger pieces of fruit into bite-sized squares, about 1-inch
(younger kids will need adult supervision or assistance when handling
a knife). Dice cheese into small cubes (or buy already cubed cheese).

The amount of fruit and cheese needed depends on how many kabobs
you are making. It will require about 5 or 6 pieces to fill each kabob.

Thread the pieces of fruit and cheese onto each wooden kabob stick
by poking them in the center with the stick. To make the kabobs more
colorful, alternate with different types of fruit and cheese as you go.
Serve the fruit and cheese kabobs immediately or chilled with a side of
plain yogurt for dipping fun. A typical serving will be two kabobs.

Safety Warning: If the fruit and cheese kabobs are being served to younger
children, prevent injury by serving them on a bendable straw instead of a wooden
skewer. Use the kabob stick to poke a hole in each piece and then string them onto
a bendable straw.

Whole grapes may pose a choking hazard for smaller children. Please eliminate
them from the recipe or chop them into small pieces before serving to kids under
3 years old.

cheesy cone

Serves 1

1 plain ice cream cone
1 romaine lettuce leaf, washed
1 ice cream scoop of low-fat cottage cheese
¼ cup dried fruit (like pineapple, cherries, or raisins), diced in
    small pieces

➤ Wrap the lettuce leaf inside the cone. Scoop the cottage cheese into the cone and sprinkle the bits of dried fruit on top to decorate. Serve immediately.

KID CREATIONS

KID CREATIONS

peanut butter quesadilla

Serves 1

1 flour tortilla
2 tablespoons peanut butter
2 tablespoons all-fruit spread

➤ Spread one-half of the tortilla with peanut butter. Fold the tortilla in half so that the filling is on the inside. Warm the quesadilla in the microwave for 30 seconds, or until warmed through. Slice it into wedges and serve with a side of all-fruit spread for dipping.

breakfast fruit wrap

(Courtesy of American Institute for Cancer Research, www.aicr.org)

Serves 1

1 tortilla, preferably whole wheat
2 teaspoons all-fruit strawberry preserves
2 tablespoons reduced-fat ricotta cheese
½ cup sliced fresh strawberries
2 tablespoons sliced almonds, toasted

➤ On a flat surface, spread strawberry preserves on tortilla. Top with ricotta cheese. Carefully top with sliced fruit and sprinkle with sliced almonds. Starting from one end, rolling tightly. Wrap in foil for neater eating.

Note: As an alternative, try replacing the strawberry preserves and strawberries with apricot preserves and sliced fresh or canned, well-drained peaches.

KID CREATIONS

turkey, spinach, and apple wrap

(Courtesy of American Institute for Cancer Research, www.aicr.org)

Serves 2

> 1 tablespoon reduced-fat mayonnaise
> 2 teaspoons honey mustard
> 2 whole-wheat flatbread wraps or flour tortillas
> 2 cups (washed and dried) baby spinach leaves, loosely packed,
>   or two large leaves soft, leafy green lettuce
> 4 thin slices turkey breast (about 4 ounces)
> ¼ Granny Smith apple, sliced paper-thin

➤ Combine mayonnaise and mustard. Lay out both wraps. Spread the edges of each with the mayonnaise mixture. Leaving a margin free on the side closest to you, arrange a layer of greens on top of the wraps. Top each layer with half the turkey. Evenly divide the apple slices and lay them lengthwise across the turkey. Fold over the end of the wrap closest to you, then fold the two sides. Roll the wrap as tightly as possible toward the opposite side. Cover each wrap tightly in plastic wrap and refrigerate, seam side down, for up to 4 hours before serving. When ready to serve, remove plastic wrap and cut each wrap in half, at an angle.

Chapter 5

TIPS ON EATING AT HOME
AND DINING OUT • • • • • • • • • • •

CHANGES IN YOUR FAMILY'S health and weight loss or weight management are affected by making small, deliberate changes to five main areas associated with their eating habits:

1. Choosing healthier snacks

2. Watching portion sizes

3. Consuming less sugar, fat, and calories

4. Eating more fruits and vegetables

5. Eating healthy meals together as a family

In the next few pages, we will provide you with helpful tips on how to eat healthy and make wise food choices, whether your family is eating at home or dining out.

Tips from the top!

"Frequency of family meals was associated with increased intake of fruits, vegetables, grains, and calcium-rich foods and negatively associated with soft drink consumption. Family meals have also been shown to contribute to the development of regular eating habits and positive psychosocial development."

—Spear, Bonnie A. "The need for family meals." *Journal of the American Dietetic Association*. Feb 2006; 106(2): 218–19.

Think About It
The Family that Eats Together . . .
Getting Back to Family Meals

As rushed as dinnertime is for most households, it is important in developing smart eating habits and fostering family bonding. Evening family mealtime
involves so much more than simply sitting at the same table consuming food.
Dinner is often the only time when the whole family eats together and when kids
can witness their parents eating and enjoying a variety of healthy foods. Gather-
ing around the table as a family allows parents to serve as positive role models
and provide a supportive environment to promote healthy eating. What you say
to your kids about healthy eating and what you offer them to eat is only a part
of what helps your kids to succeed in their quest for healthy eating. The best
motivator for kids to eat and be healthy is seeing their parents living and eating
healthy alongside them!

Another bonus to family meals is that some of the best discussions between
parents and children happen around the dinner table. When families sit down
together at the table and take a break from distractions like televisions and tele-
phones, they find valuable time to simply focus on each other. Bonding and building open communication with your kids are also important steps in developing
stronger, healthier children and families.

Try these tips when planning your family meals at home:

* *Make the whole meal a family affair, from planning to cleanup.* Include your
  kids in the process of meal planning, grocery shopping, meal preparation,
  table setting, and cleaning up . . . not just the eating! The more involved
  they are in the process, the more they learn about making healthy choices. It

also makes the work associated with dinnertime less of a burden because the tasks are shared and it shows that making the effort as a family is important.

* *Multitask when preparing ingredients.* Some days you may have more time and energy to dice and cook than others. Take advantage of those moments and make ingredients that can be used for more than one meal. For instance, it doesn't add much more work to cook six chicken breasts on the grill instead of making just four. Grill the extras at the same time, then freeze them for later. When you need a quick meal, chop them up and use them for fajitas or chicken salad the next day.

* *Keep your meals simple and realistic.* It may be a fun idea to plan an occasional fancy family meal, but quick and easy meals actually make it to the table a lot more often than labor-intensive and costly ones. Keep in mind your family's busy schedules, likes and dislikes, and budget when deciding on your meals. Instead of planning recipes that call for a lot of items or obscure ingredients, focus on recipes that use staple ingredients and can be prepared and set on the table in less than an hour.

* *Let meals appeal to your family's senses.* Think about providing pleasing aromas, varieties in color and texture, and interesting plate arrangements when preparing and serving meals. Details like these don't add much time to the process but can go a long way in making food (especially new healthy options) more appealing to kids and adults!

KEEPING YOUR FAMILY'S FOOD SAFE TO EAT

Plan ahead to defrost the meat you will need for dinner. Don't defrost food on the kitchen counter at room temperature. A great amount of bacteria grows in the 40 to 100°F range. Room temperature falls into that range. For this same reason, it isn't even wise to leave meat at room temperature for more than an hour. Instead, thaw meat in the refrigerator, immerse an air-tight package of meat in cold tap water (as long as you change the water every 30 minutes), or defrost the meat in the microwave.

If you place raw meat, poultry, or seafood in the refrigerator, always store it on the bottom shelf and place it in a tray or on a plate to prevent dripping. Food placed on higher shelves may drip juices and bacteria onto other foods as they begin to thaw.

Don't wash or rinse meat or poultry before cooking it. Although we often equate rinsing foods with cleanliness, the USDA's Meat and Poultry Helpline (see Resources) reports that this can actually cause more harm than good. Bacteria from rinsed meat and poultry spread to the sink, faucet, your hands, and anything else you touch or that comes in contact with the raw meat. Even more contamination takes place if you then place other foods (like fresh fruits or vegetables) into the sink. Bacteria found on the meat is destroyed during cooking, but bacteria that gathers on items like salad ingredients will likely be served to your family and dinner guests.

Wash fruits and vegetables before eating, especially if they will be served without further cooking. Rinsing your produce under cold water removes any dirt and reduces the amount of bacteria that may be present on the surface. If food items have a hard peel (like potatoes) you can also scrub the surface with a brush to clean it further. Do not use soap or detergent when cleaning fruits and vegetables. See the box on page 127 for tips on washing fruits and vegetables with lemon juice.

The acid from lemon juice can help rid your fruits and vegetables of bacteria. Here's how to make your own homemade lemon juice wash:

1. Cut a lemon in half and squeeze the juice into a bowl.

2. Measure 2 tablespoons of the lemon juice in the bowl into a liquid measuring cup. Add 2 tablespoons of distilled white vinegar, 2 tablespoons of baking soda, and 1 cup of water. Stir well until the baking soda is completely dissolved.

3. Pour the lemon juice mixture into a clean spray bottle.

4. Place your fruits and vegetables in a colander and spray them generously with the lemon juice wash. Let the sprayed produce sit for 5 to 10 minutes and then rinse with cool water.

Clean as you go. Wash utensils, knives, cutting boards, and counters with hot soapy water right after using them. Bacteria are easily passed by reusing unclean items. Do not move on to the preparation of the next food item on an unclean surface or use the unwashed utensils for another food item. Also, wash your hands often with warm water and soap when preparing and cooking food to reduce cross-contamination.

Make sure that the food is cooked all the way through before serving it. Cut into the middle of meat and poultry to ensure that it is thoroughly cooked. Also, avoid serving your family raw or partially cooked eggs or any food items that contain raw eggs.

Take care of leftovers and perishable foods promptly. Do not leave perishable items sitting out after using them. It is too easy to lose track of how long they have been kept unrefrigerated. Also, freeze or refrigerate your leftovers as soon as you are done eating, or once they cool, to avoid them spoiling. To ensure that food is eaten in a timely manner, it's also helpful to label the container or freezer bag with the date on which the meal was made.

Psst... *Parents*

Making Wiser Food Choices

Cutting down on fat and excess calories doesn't always have to involve drastic changes. It's about making smarter choices and practicing moderation, not deprivation. Making small, deliberate adjustments to old eating habits can yield positive results for your family.

* Enjoy food, but eat less of it. Oversized portions and too many second helpings of favorite foods add up quickly.

* Use a cooking spray instead of using oils when you sauté foods.

* Pay attention to food labels when deciding which products to buy.

* Skip the heavy dressings and cheeses in your salads and pile on the beans and peas instead.

* Bake or grill foods instead of frying them.

* Cut down on soda and other sugar-sweetened drinks. Replace them with water, 100% juice, or seltzer (choose a sodium-free and aspartame-free option).

* Choose lean cuts of meat and trim visible fat from your meats or remove the skin from poultry before cooking them.

* Only allow kids to eat snacks in certain places, like in the kitchen, where distractions are minimal. Keeping snack time away from the television or computer will save your child countless calories from mindless munching.

* Start kids with a small portion. They should eat smaller portions than adults. They can always ask for seconds if they are still hungry.

* Reduce the number of snacks your child eats each day. Kids who snack often tend to fill up and then not eat their meals as well. Scheduled snack times will help monitor how much and what she or he eats and will help kids learn structure for eating.

* Save treats and sweets for special occasions and resist the urge to use them as rewards for kids. Instead, keep food completely out of the punishment and reward system and use affection and nonfood items as incentives for kids.

* Resist the urge to revert to their favorites. Variety promotes optimal nutrition in kids. As parents, we tend to offer the healthy choices we know our kids will eat, like carrots and apples, but often neglect other healthy foods they may have enjoyed in the past or might like if they were to try them.

Money Smart Tips for Buying and Using Fresh Fruits and Vegetables

* *Buy your fruits and vegetables in small quantities.* There are many fresh fruits and vegetables that don't last for very long. By purchasing smaller amounts, you will have as much as your family can eat before they go bad, without having to waste money and food by throwing away overripe or spoiled items.

* *Remember to keep it simple.* Ready-to-eat foods like those that are pre-washed or pre-cut are convenient, but they also cost more. Stick to buying fruits and vegetables in their simplest form to save on your budget. Instead, take the extra time at home to wash, cut, and portion out your produce at home after purchasing it.

* *Use leftovers and overripe produce for cooking and baking whenever possible.* Add leftover vegetables to soups, casseroles, and other dishes. Also, fruit that is getting too ripe to eat on its own may still work nicely in baked goods and blended drinks, such as bananas for muffins or berries for making smoothies.

* *Celebrate the seasons with your produce!* Learn which fruits and vegetables are in season and use them more often during that time of year. Fruits and vegetables will be more affordable, easier to find, and more flavorful when they are in their prime season. Check out your local farmers' markets and farm stands to discover which produce items are in season.

* *Grow your own fruits and vegetables.* Plant a small kitchen garden in your yard or grow a few favorite items in pots on the deck to give your family an easily accessible source for fresh and unprocessed produce. A few easy-to-grow choices for beginning gardeners include tomatoes, cucumbers, and herbs. Be sure to include your kids in the process, too!

✦ KIDS' CORNER • • • • • • • • • • • • • • • • • •

Hey, kids! If you're reading this, or if someone is reading it to you, then you're getting ready to make some changes for a healthier life. Good for you!

We want to remind you to be safe and smart while you're getting healthy. You are much more important than your size or your weight. Drastic weight loss plans and diets may seem like the answer to all your problems because they seem to work fast and don't involve a lot of work. *Don't fall for the hype.* These types of weight loss programs can hurt your health. Skipping meals, eating only one or two specific foods for days, making yourself vomit after you eat, taking laxatives, and drinking mixes or popping pills to curb your appetite are *not* going to make you thin and healthy. Methods like those may cause you to lose weight, but they will also leave you feeling hungry and will make you sick. This bears repeating. *You are more important than your weight.*

Remember, it took months or possibly years for you to gain the extra pounds you're now trying to lose. It will take some time to lose them again. But by making small, smart changes to your daily eating and exercise habits, you will lose the weight, still feel satisfied at the end of the day, and grow stronger and healthier.

Here are a few changes you can make on your own to help in your weight loss:

✶ *Eat breakfast even if you don't feel like it.* Skipping breakfast often leads to overeating later in the day. If you're a light morning eater, try a breakfast shake, a piece of fruit, or a container of yogurt, but start the day right by putting something nutritious in your body.

✶ *When you do go out for fast food, say "no" to super-sized meals.* Many fast food portions are bigger and packed with more calories, fat, and sodium than what you should consume in a meal. You don't need to make them even bigger by ordering a super-sized meal. You can still eat fast foods occasionally, but remember that moderation and self-control are important. Order a regular-sized sandwich, a small order of French fries or a side salad, and a small drink such as water, milk, or juice. If you do order a big meal, split it with a friend or family member.

✶ *Think before you drink.* How many sodas or sugary drinks do you consume every day? They may taste good but they are loaded with empty calories, sugars, and other ingredients that do nothing more than fill your body with extra junk it doesn't need! Get rid of them or at least cut down. Start by replacing one soda each day with a bottle of water.

DINING OUT SMARTER

When you're planning meals for your family at home it is much easier to adhere to a healthy eating plan and monitor how well everyone is eating. Eating out at restaurants presents a new set of challenges, but it can still be done!

Below are some suggestions to help you and the whole family make healthy eating choices while dining out:

* *Start the meal by ordering salads that are packed with vegetables for the whole family* . It will help control hunger and help your family feel satisfied sooner.

* *If entrees are big, ask for an extra plate and split them with another family member.* Remember, it's not always necessary for your child to clean his plate as long as he has eaten a balanced and filling meal. It's also fine to ask your waiter to box up some of the meal and take leftovers home with you.

* *Ask your waiter how the foods are prepared so that your family can make wise selections from the menu.* There is nothing wrong with asking questions about whether the meal is deep-fried, grilled, or baked. Try to stick with meals that are blackened, grilled, broiled, baked, boiled, or stir-fried.

* *Understand that it's acceptable to ask for sauce, gravy, and spreads to be left off from meals or placed on the side so that the amount can be monitored.* The same principle applies when ordering salads. Asking for dressings or sauces on the side makes it easier to control portions. A little can go a long way with fatty or calorie-laden toppings.

* *Order menu items instead of the all-you-can-eat buffet.* There is a much greater chance of overeating and losing sight of portion control when family members are loading their plates at the buffet and can make multiple trips to refill.

* *If your family splurges for dessert when dining out, try to order a fruit-based dessert or split the dessert into smaller portions.* It's not necessary to ban all desserts. Instead, simply reduce how often and how much of them your kids eat.

PART III

$\bullet\ \bullet$

EXERCISE

Chapter 6

FITNESS BASICS FOR HEALTHY, ACTIVE KIDS • • • • • • •

JUST LIKE ADULTS, KIDS need regular physical activity to stay healthy, both physically and mentally. Regular exercise promotes and controls a healthy body weight; builds stronger bones, joints, and muscle strength; improves flexibility; provides more energy; boosts self-confidence; improves concentration at school and home; develops motor skills; and increases the child's ability to handle stress. Teaching your child the importance of fitness and how to incorporate physical activity into his or her daily life now will reap rewards for years to come.

HOW MUCH IS ENOUGH?

As a general rule, children should participate in at least sixty minutes of physical activity every day. However, helping your kids meet those recommendations isn't as simple as sending them outside to play for an hour or so. Kids often do activities in short bursts, which may not technically be long enough to give them a true workout. Although it is possible that some children can be physically active on their own, getting them involved in structured exercises, group activities, and games, as well as individual or team sports, are excellent ways to help them meet their physical fitness requirements.

Kids will usually get some exercise during their school day from recess and physical education classes, but it is best not to rely on that as their only daily exercise. Many busy school schedules no longer allow for daily recesses and gym classes for students, especially for those in the higher grades. Getting the whole family involved in physical activities—that means you too, parents!—is the best way to ensure that your kids are getting the exercise they need every day.

While you might think that it will be tough to keep kids active for an hour, it's important to remember that the recommendation is for sixty minutes of physical activity every day. It does not necessarily have to been done all at one time, as long as the exercise is broken up into segments that last long enough to give kids a true workout. Physical activities that last around 15 to 20 minutes usually work well, depending on the intensity of the exercise.

Here are some examples of how your child could fit an hour of physical activity into an average day without much extra strain on a busy schedule:

* ★ Set the alarm for 15 minutes earlier and start the morning with a short routine of structured exercises like sit-ups, jumping jacks, and stretches to get the whole family awake and moving.

* ★ Have your child walk or ride his bike to and from school, if it's feasible.

* ★ Later on, engage in a quick game of tag or basketball with family and friends in the backyard, or take a family bike ride.

Think About It

As a parent, you hold a lot of influence when it comes to shaping your kid's attitudes and views on physical activity. Like it or not, the way you view exercise and the value you place on it will affect your child.

Here are a few tips to keep in mind when encouraging physical activity for the whole family:

* Be a positive example for your family by leading an active lifestyle yourself and keeping a good attitude while doing it!

* Provide your kids with equipment that encourages physical movement over sedentary activities. Some examples include bicycles, rollerblades, balls, baseball gloves and bats, tennis racquets, basketball hoop, a swing set, or other backyard playground equipment.

* Make frequent trips with your kids to places that promote being active, like parks or ball fields.

* Find ways to incorporate physical activity into your family's routine. Take family bike rides, walks, runs, hikes, or simply play active games together.

* Remember to keep physical activity fun! If you want your family to stick to it, they need to enjoy it, so find ways to be active that your kids like doing.

* Encourage your child to try new individual and team sports and be supportive when she shows an interest in one.

* Keep safety at the forefront. Discuss safety precautions with your child, provide protective gear like helmets and wrist pads or knee pads for kids, and be sure that the activities are age-appropriate.

Tips from the top!

KEEPING KIDS MOTIVATED AT ANY AGE

Encouraging kids to get out and exercise can be tough, but guiding them toward age-appropriate activities will help get them excited, and stay motivated, to be active.

Here is some age-based advice from KidsHealth (www.kidshealth.org):

Preschoolers: Preschoolers need play and exercise that helps them continue to develop important motor skills—kicking or throwing a ball, playing tag or follow the leader, hopping on one foot, riding a trike or bike with training wheels, freeze dancing, or running obstacle courses.

Although some sports leagues may be open to kids as young as 4, organized and team sports are not recommended until they're a little older. Preschoolers can't understand complex rules and often lack the attention span, skills, and coordination needed to play sports. Instead of learning to play a sport, they should work on fundamental skills.

School-age: With school-age kids spending more time on sedentary pursuits like watching TV and playing computer games, the challenge for parents is to help them find physical activities they enjoy and feel successful doing. These can range from traditional sports like baseball and basketball to martial arts, biking, hiking, and playing outside.

As kids learn basic skills and simple rules in the early school-age years, there might only be a few athletic standouts. As kids get older, differences in ability and personality become more apparent. Commitment and interest level often go along with ability, which is why it's important to find an activity that's right for your child. Schedules start getting busy during these years, but don't forget to set aside some time for free play.

Teenagers: Teens have many choices when it comes to being active—from school sports to after-school interests, such as yoga or skateboarding. It's important to remember that physical activity must be planned and often has to be sandwiched between various responsibilities and commitments.

Do what you can to make it easy for your teen to exercise by providing transportation and the necessary gear or equipment (including workout clothes). In some cases, the right clothes and shoes might help a shy teen feel comfortable biking or going to the gym.

© 1995–2012 . *The Nemours Foundation/KidsHealth®. Reprinted with permission.*
http://kidshealth.org/parent/nutrition_center/staying_fit/active_kids.html#

THE BEST TYPES OF EXERCISE FOR KIDS

The Physical Activity Guidelines for American children and adolescents established by the United States Department of Health and Human Services encourage a focus on three types of activity:

1. Aerobic
2. Muscle-strengthening
3. Bone-strengthening

Aerobic activities get kids to rhythmically move their large muscles for prolonged periods, which is helpful in increasing cardiorespiratory fitness. Cardiorespiratory fitness is the body's ability to transport oxygen to the muscles during extended exercise and the ability of the muscles to absorb and use the oxygen while exercising. Activities like running, jumping rope, dancing, and bicycling are examples of aerobic activities.

Muscle-strengthening activities require muscles to do more work than they do during regular daily activities. This excess work, also known as overload, strengthens the muscles used by the child for the activity. Activities for muscle-strengthening may be structured, such as using resistance bands, performing sit-ups and pull-ups, or lifting weights. They can also be unstructured and incorporated as play, such as climbing trees, playing tug-of-war, or using playground equipment.

Bone-strengthening activities create force on the child's bones to promote bone growth and strength. The force is commonly produced by some sort of impact with the ground. A few common examples of activities that strengthen bones include playing basketball and tennis, running, playing hopscotch, or jumping rope. Bone-strengthening activities are often also aerobic and/or muscle-strengthening.

We also recommend including exercises and activities that promote agility and flexibility into your child's routine.

Agility-boosting activities improve the body's ability to change directions in an effective manner. Agility requires a combination of balance, speed, strength, and coordination. Activities and exercises that work on a kid's agility focus on ways to build on each of those elements. A few examples of agility-boosting activities include jumping jacks, shuffle running, and ladder drills, which we will explain in further detail in Chapter 7.

Flexibility-boosting activities encourage your child's joints and muscles to move through a full range of motion. Flexibility allows for more movement around the joints and helps create better posture, reduces risk of injuries, and lessens muscle soreness and cramping. Many exercises that help with flexibility also leave the child's mind and body feeling more relaxed. Activities that promote flexibility generally include a variety of stretches like forward bends, calf stretches, and torso twists. These stretches, and others, will be discussed and demonstrated in Chapter 7.

YOUR CHILD'S HEART RATE AND PHYSICAL ACTIVITY

First of all, what is heart rate? Heart rate is simply the average number of times per minute the heart beats—or pumps blood—through your child's body.

What is the normal heart rate for kids when they are not exercising, or at rest?

Age	Beats Per Minute (BPM)
Babies to Age 1	100–160
Ages 1 to 10	60–140
Ages 10 to Adults	60–100

Since the average resting heart rate varies with age and for each individual, the heart rate during exercise will vary also. On the average, a 4-year-old should have an exercising heart rate of around 137 beats per minute. By 5 to 7 years old, the average heart rate during activity will be closer to 133 beats per minute. It lowers to an average 130 beats per minute for 8- to 11-year-olds. By the time kids reach adolescence, the exercising heart rate is significantly lower, at 115 beats per minute.

⚡ QUICK DRILL

You'll learn what is normal for your child over time. The best way to do this is to record your child's resting heart rate and then monitor it over the course of the physical activity. For example, take your child to the park to play on the playground equipment. Start by taking her or his resting heart rate, then let her or him run around for about 10 minutes and take her or his pulse again. Let her or him return to playing and check her or his heart rate every 10 minutes. Record the results. This will give you a fair understanding of what are normal resting and active heart rates for your child.

To see if kids are exerting themselves enough during physical activity you can do a quick pulse check. Here's how:

1. Use your index, middle, and ring fingers and place them on the child's wrist right below the base of the thumb. You can also take the pulse on one side of the windpipe.

2. Press slightly until you can feel the blood pulsing.

3. Use a watch or clock that has a second hand and time 10 seconds.

4. Count the number of times your child's heart beats (each time it pulses) during those 10 seconds and then multiple it by six to calculate his or her heart rate.

If you notice that your child's heart rate is on the low end during physical activity, encourage her or him to play harder. Maybe challenging her or him to race across the field will get that heart rate up! Conversely, if you notice that her or his heart rate is on the higher end, encourage him to take more frequent breaks to talk, rest, or grab a drink of water.

SUPER STRUCTURED ACTIVITIES TO GET KIDS MOVING

We recommend including these structured activities in your child's fitness plan. Please refer to Chapter 7 of this book to find explanations and step-by-step demonstrations of each activity.

* Standing Incline Push-Up (page 154)
* High Bar Pull-Up (page 155)
* High Bar Chin-Up (page 156)
* Monkey Bar Arm Walk (page 157)
* Triceps Dips (page 158)
* Balance Beam Step-Up (page 159)
* Balance Beam Squats (page 160)
* Jumping Jacks (page 161)
* Running Ladder Drills (page 162)
* Backward Running (page 163)
* Running in Place with High Knees (page 164)
* Shuffle Running (page 165)
* Burpees (page 166)
* Mountain Climbers (page 167)
* Standing Forward-Bend Toe Touches (page 168)
* Seated Torso Twist with Leg Cross-Over (page 169)
* Butterfly Stretch (page 170)
* Child's Pose (page 171)
* Standing Quadriceps Stretch (page 172)
* Shoulder Stretch (page 173)
* Standing Calf Stretch (page 174)

FUN UNSTRUCTURED ACTIVITIES TO ENJOY OUTDOORS

We recommend incorporating these unstructured activities in your child's exercise routine. Please refer to Chapter 8 of this book to find explanations and helpful suggestions about each activity.

* Biking (page 176)
* Jumping Rope (page 177)
* Skateboarding (page 178)
* Inline Skating (page 178)
* Swimming (page 178)
* Tag (page 178)
* Two-Square or Four-Square (page 179)
* Dodgeball (page 180)
* Hide and Seek (page 180)
* Backwards Baseball (page 181)
* Basketball (page 182)
* Soccer (page 182)
* Hiking (page 183)
* Frisbee
* Catch (baseball or football)

Safety from Head to Toe!

Not only is the health of your child important to us, but so is his or her safety! Did you know that not using protective equipment, using the wrong gear, or wearing equipment that doesn't fit properly are major causes of injury among kids?

Keep these tips in mind when providing your child with protective gear:

1. **Protect the head.** Teach your kids to wear a helmet when participating in sports like biking, skateboarding, skating, skiing, hockey, football, baseball, and softball.

   ✓ Make sure the helmet is intended for the sport your child is playing. Not all helmets are made for use with all activities.

   ✓ Look for the sticker on bike helmets that says they meet the safety standard set by the Consumer Product Safety Commission (CPSC), a federal agency that creates safety standards for bike helmets and other safety equipment.

   ✓ Check for fit on your child's head. The helmet should fit snugly, but feel comfortable on his or her head, and it should not tilt backward or forward.

2. **The eyes have it!** A lot of sports, especially those that include balls or other flying objects, put kids' eyes at risk. Insist that she or he wear protective eye gear.

   ✓ Facemasks or helmet shields should be worn when the child participates in sports like ice hockey or football. They should also be used by the batter and catcher when playing softball and baseball.

   ✓ Goggles are recommended for kids when they are playing racquetball, tennis, snowboarding, street hockey, or skiing.

   ✓ A child who wears glasses and plays active sports should be fitted for prescription polycarbonate goggles. Regular glasses break easily and do not offer the same amount of protection.

   ✓ Eye protection should fit securely on the child's face. For your child's comfort, make sure it also has cushions that rest above the eyebrows and over the nose.

3. Guard the mouth. A child's mouth is very sensitive. Mouth guards should be worn to protect your child's mouth, teeth, and tongue.

✓ Children should wear mouth guards when engaging in contact sports like martial arts, boxing, or wrestling. Mouth guards are also recommended when playing other types of sports where head injuries are a greater risk, such as football and hockey.

✓ You can buy mouth guards that adjust to the size of your child's mouth at your local sports store, or have her or him fitted for one by a dentist.

✓ To protect against accidental breakage or injury to the child, orthodontic retainers should be removed before your child plays, exercises, or participates in sports.

4. Protect the knees, elbows, and wrists, too! Wearing guards on the elbows and wrists when engaging in activities and contact sports can prevent arm and wrist fractures. Knee, shin, shoulder, and thigh pads help protect your child from ugly breaks, scrapes, and bruises.

✓ Insist that kids wear guards on their knees, elbows, and wrists to protect against falls when riding scooters, skateboards, or when inline skating.

✓ Provide your child with guards or pads to use when playing sports like hockey, football, and martial arts.

✓ If you are unsure of the proper pads or guards your child should wear for a particular sport, check with the child's coach or doctor.

5. Keep kids safe all the way down to their feet. Equipping your child with the proper footwear will cut down on unnecessary trips and falls.

✓ Some sports, like football, soccer, baseball, and softball, require cleats to maintain surefootedness on the field. Other sports, such as skateboarding, require special shoes for safety, too. Check with your child's coach to find out what shoes will work best.

✓ Athletic shoes that are worn out do not lend proper support or traction. Replace your child's shoes and cleats often to keep his or her feet safe.

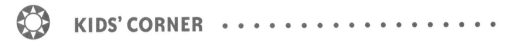

KIDS' CORNER

Here are some simple ways to add exercise to your daily schedule:

★ *Hit the road!* Instead of asking your parents to drive you, put your feet to good use. Walk, ride your bike, or inline skate to places that are nearby whenever it's possible. You'll save gas, enjoy some fresh air, and get a few minutes of aerobic exercise all at the same time. Don't forget to ask your parents for permission first and always tell them where you are going!

★ *Get into the swing of things.* When you do walk, get your arms into it, too! The arm motions help you keep a quick pace and also give your arms and legs a little workout.

★ *Become a stair master.* Instead of hopping onto an elevator when the opportunity arises, choose to take the stairs. Your legs, knees, and cardiovascular system will benefit from the decision.

★ *Jam out while doing your chores.* Okay, so we know you probably don't like to do your chores around the house, but they still need to be done. Why not add some fun to them and get some exercise at the same time? Crank up your favorite tunes, and dance your way through chores. The job will seem to get done faster, and your body and mood will get a boost!

Chapter 7

EASY DOES IT! · · · · · · · · · · · · ·
(Fun Timed Activities)

FAMILIES THAT BEGIN INTEGRATING fun exercise into their lives tend to take on healthier lifestyles. Whether it's because they become more mindful or more aware, when kids get to know their bodies, they become more conscious of how their bodies perform and how exercise will affect their performance. They also learn about discipline and commitment, which are huge life lessons.

There are three areas of fitness that will help improve overall health: strength, speed, and flexibility. In the following pages, you will find fun activities that you can do as a family to target these aspects of fitness.

Strength training isn't only for adults and it's certainly not just about lifting weights. Kids can greatly benefit from performing bodyweight exercises. While on the outside we see our children laughing and having fun while exercising, what's going on inside—particularly within their central nervous system—is profound. When kids begin strength training early on, they tend to possess elevated levels of body control, muscle response, and internal balance throughout the rest of their lives. Additionally, they typically enjoy higher self-esteem and confidence, and gravitate toward goal-orientated thinking.

Strength training also supports muscle growth by shocking the muscle tissue and pushing the body to become stronger, faster, and more agile. Bringing the kids to the park or gym for bodyweight training is a great way to get their muscles and cardiovascular systems in tip-top shape.

Kids shouldn't be overly concerned with aesthetics and trying to fit the "standard" mold of what magazines and television exhibit. In *Combat Fat for Kids!*, we're concerned with conditioning kids so that they are receiving enough exercise to control body composition levels (body fat percentage versus lean muscle tissue). When kids focus on moving, they will naturally burn calories. When they lift, carry, and manipulate their body weight, this will naturally build muscle, stronger bones, and connective tissue. If we can teach kids to stay the course, they will grow into healthier adults, both physically and emotionally.

Speed is important for many reasons, especially for kids. Working with your children to increase their speed will help them to utilize that speed in becoming more active, and ultimately, healthier kids and adults. Integrating different types of speed-focused exercises into your family's fitness routine also helps to promote safety during physical activity. The faster you can react to something, the safer you are, whether it is avoiding a fall or responding to someone in need.

There are many applications for speed, whether it's assisting your children to perform better during their favorite activity or sport, or giving their bodies a helping hand when they're adapting to proper movement mechanics and motor skills. Speed and agility training is all about avoiding injury, running the ball down the field faster, and beating Dad on a dash to the other end of the yard.

Flexibility is simply a means to allow joints to move over a full range of motion. The act of performing bodyweight exercises is not just about building strength; they are also natural flexibility exercises. Dynamic stretches, in which you maintain motion rather than holding a static stretch, are a more natural kid-based movement.

WORKOUT ROUTINE SCHEDULE

This is a three-day workout routine schedule. You can also add more workout days as needed. If adding additional workout days, choose any four exercises from each fitness area for each day.

For each workout day, follow these steps:

1. Perform the exercises marked in each fitness area for that day.

2. With Jungle Gym Strength, complete three sets of 10 repetitions.

3. With Cheetah-Like Speed, complete three sets of 30 to 60 seconds for each exercise.

4. With Cat-Like Flexibility, complete three sets of 15 to 30 second holds for each exercise.

Jungle gym strength: Simple bodyweight strength exercises using playground equipment.

Cheetah-like speed: Fun cardio drills and races incorporating work-to-rest ratio concepts (see box below).

Cat-like flexibility: Simple yoga-inspired stretches and flexibility exercises to improve range of motion and mobility.

Psst... *Parents*
Work-to-Rest Ratio

Work-to-rest (W-T-R) ratio is a means to keep tabs on the amount of time a person is performing a specific bodyweight exercise, stretch, or speed drill. This is a great way to allow kids to work at their own fitness level, rather than counting repetitions. For all intents and purposes, we just want kids to move. For adults, W-T-R ratio is a prescribed range of work times and rest times that will elicit a specific training outcome. However, for this book we will more appropriately use various ranges to keep kids interested and motivated. In this way, we can look at the prescribed ranges as challenges for kids to conquer.

The best way to discover an appropriate W-T-R ratio for your child is to begin by setting the bar too low; in other words, start with a work time that you know they will be able to handle without a problem. When they complete that goal successfully, be sure to show them some praise for a job well done. Right off the bat, this will help them to feel confident and strong. More than likely, your child will then quite naturally ask to go to the opposite extreme, overextending themselves and learning a good life lesson in the process. When the dust clears, it will be easy to find a middle road between the two and you can then begin progressive training from there.

Note: While there is no set parameter for how much kids should rest between exercises, always remember that it is important to allow them to recover between sets and exercises, especially when first getting started. You can often tell if your kid is overexerting himself by watching his breathing. If he is breathing too heavily, make sure he takes a break. If he is experiencing difficulty performing exercises or shows any sign of discomfort, STOP! These activities are all about progressive achievement. If you want to see results and continue to progress, it's also important to keep things fresh and change your exercise routine once in a while. The body is very clever and will quickly adapt to a stagnant routine. For kids, changing things around can be as simple as giving cues such as "lift higher," "move faster," or "go lower."

JUNGLE GYM STRENGTH

Exercise List	Day 1	Day 2	Day 3
Standing Incline Push-Up (page 154)	x		x
High Bar Pull-Up (page 155)	x		x
High Bar Chin-Up (page 156)	x		
Monkey Bar Arm Walk (page 157)	x	x	
Triceps Dips (page 158)		x	x
Balance Beam Step-Up (page 159)		x	
Balance Beam Squats (page 160)		x	x

CHEETAH-LIKE SPEED

Exercise List	Day 1	Day 2	Day 3
Jumping Jacks (page 161)	x	x	
Running Ladder Drills (page 162)	x		x
Backward Running (page 163)		x	x
Running in Place with High Knees (page 164)		x	
Shuffle Running (page 165)		x	
Burpees (page 166)	x		x
Mountain Climbers (page 167)	x		x

CAT-LIKE FLEXIBILITY

Exercise List	Day 1	Day 2	Day 3
Standing Forward-Bend Toe Touches (page 168)	x		x
Seated Torso Twist with Leg Cross-Over (page 169)		x	
Butterfly Stretch (page 170)	x	x	x
Child's Pose (page 171)		x	
Standing Quadriceps Stretch (page 172)		x	
Shoulder Stretch (page 173)	x		x
Standing Calf Stretch (page 174)	x		x

Standing Incline Push-Up

Stand in front of a chest-height bar about 1 foot away, with your arms extended in front of your chest. Lean forward toward the bar and grab the bar with your hands and arms extended. Bend your elbows and bring your chest toward the bar. Extend your elbows and push your chest away from the bar.

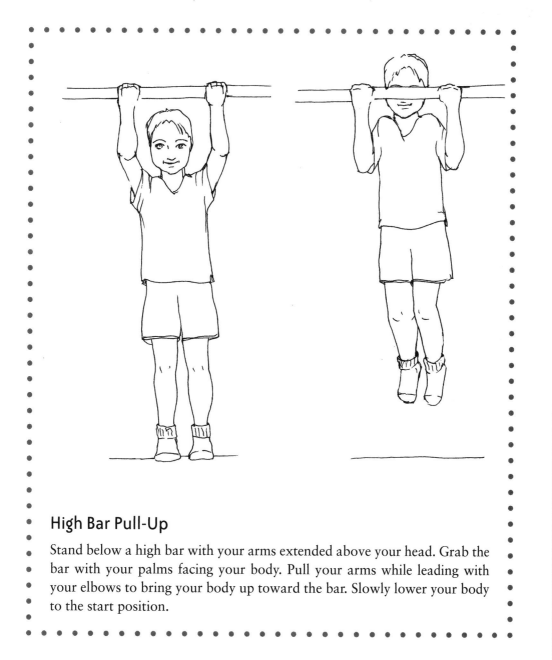

High Bar Pull-Up

Stand below a high bar with your arms extended above your head. Grab the bar with your palms facing your body. Pull your arms while leading with your elbows to bring your body up toward the bar. Slowly lower your body to the start position.

JUNGLE GYM STRENGTH

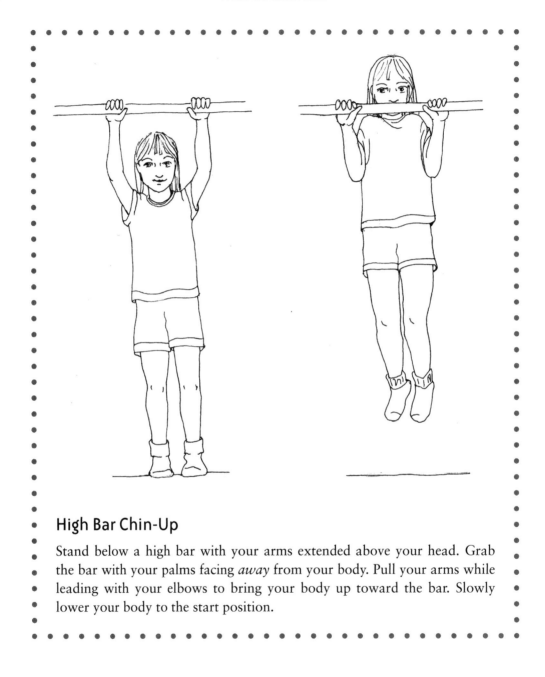

High Bar Chin-Up

Stand below a high bar with your arms extended above your head. Grab the bar with your palms facing *away* from your body. Pull your arms while leading with your elbows to bring your body up toward the bar. Slowly lower your body to the start position.

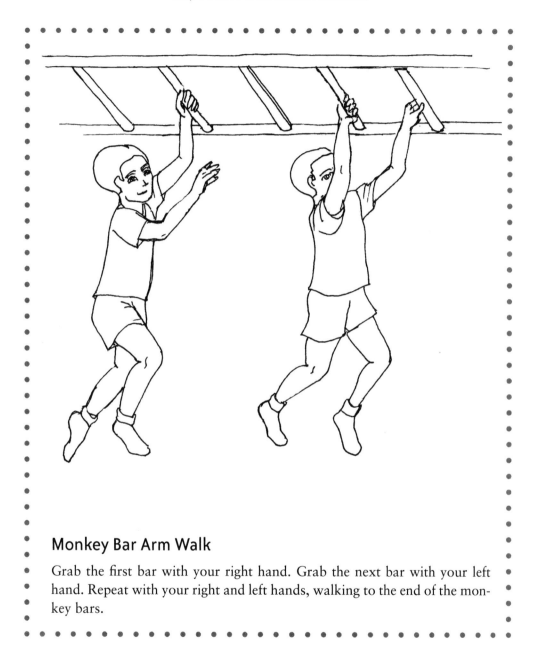

Monkey Bar Arm Walk

Grab the first bar with your right hand. Grab the next bar with your left hand. Repeat with your right and left hands, walking to the end of the monkey bars.

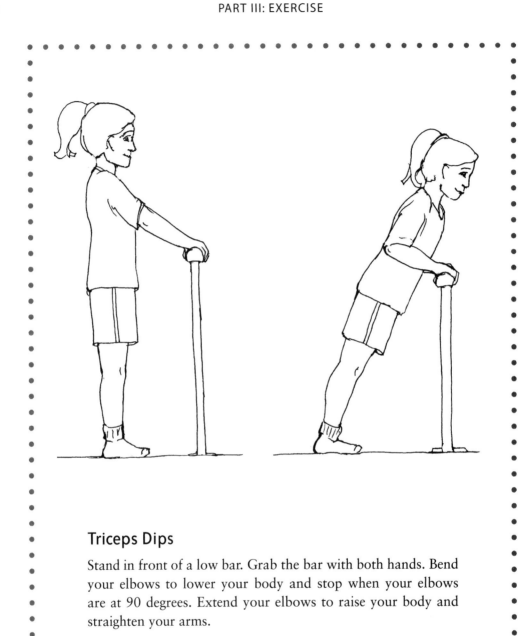

Triceps Dips

Stand in front of a low bar. Grab the bar with both hands. Bend your elbows to lower your body and stop when your elbows are at 90 degrees. Extend your elbows to raise your body and straighten your arms.

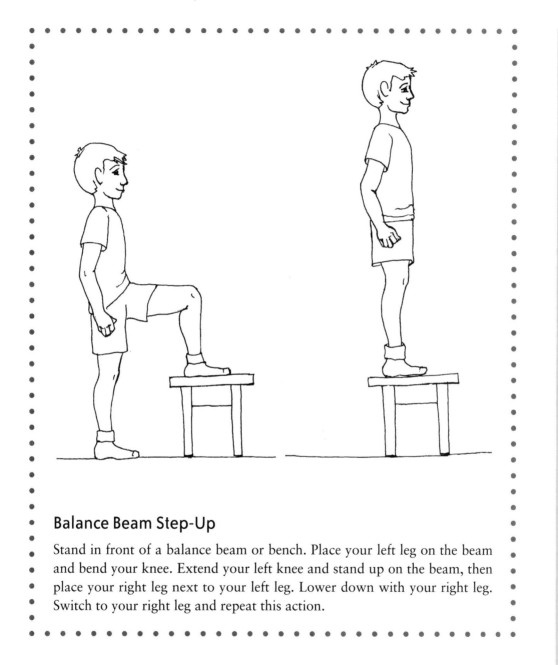

Balance Beam Step-Up

Stand in front of a balance beam or bench. Place your left leg on the beam and bend your knee. Extend your left knee and stand up on the beam, then place your right leg next to your left leg. Lower down with your right leg. Switch to your right leg and repeat this action.

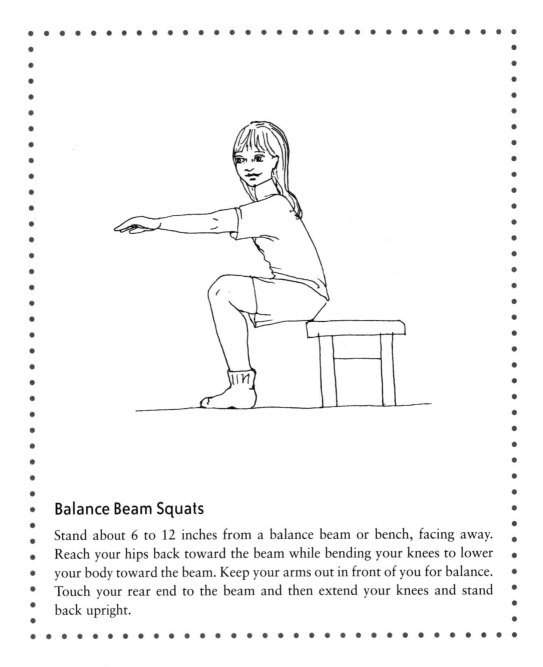

Balance Beam Squats

Stand about 6 to 12 inches from a balance beam or bench, facing away. Reach your hips back toward the beam while bending your knees to lower your body toward the beam. Keep your arms out in front of you for balance. Touch your rear end to the beam and then extend your knees and stand back upright.

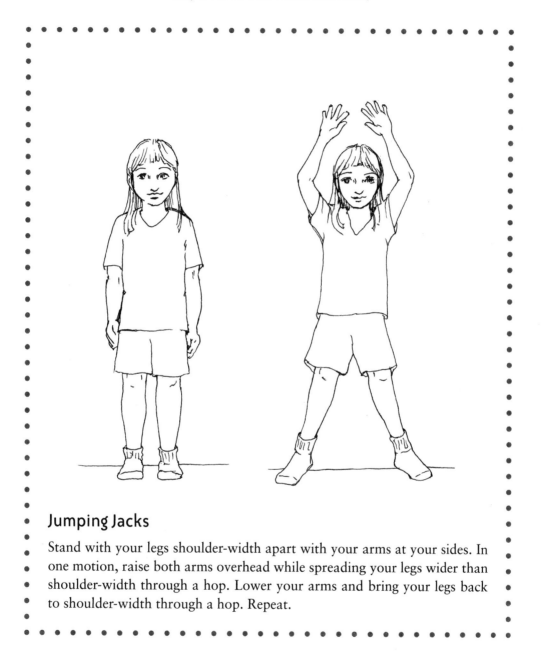

Jumping Jacks

Stand with your legs shoulder-width apart with your arms at your sides. In one motion, raise both arms overhead while spreading your legs wider than shoulder-width through a hop. Lower your arms and bring your legs back to shoulder-width through a hop. Repeat.

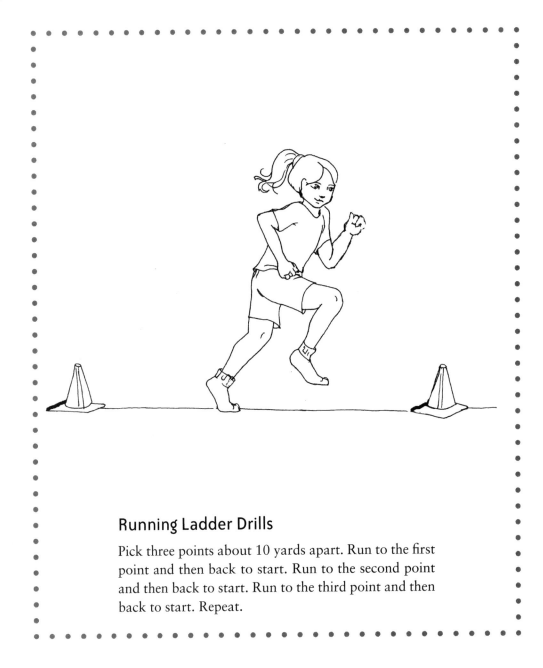

Running Ladder Drills

Pick three points about 10 yards apart. Run to the first
point and then back to start. Run to the second point
and then back to start. Run to the third point and then
back to start. Repeat.

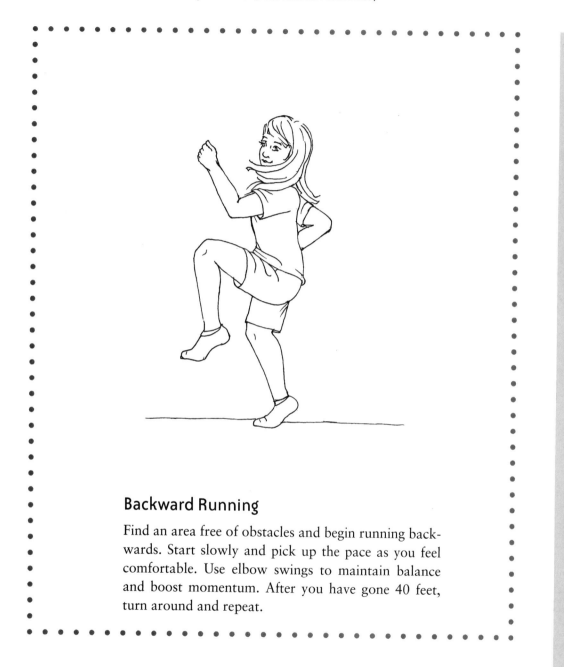

Backward Running

Find an area free of obstacles and begin running backwards. Start slowly and pick up the pace as you feel comfortable. Use elbow swings to maintain balance and boost momentum. After you have gone 40 feet, turn around and repeat.

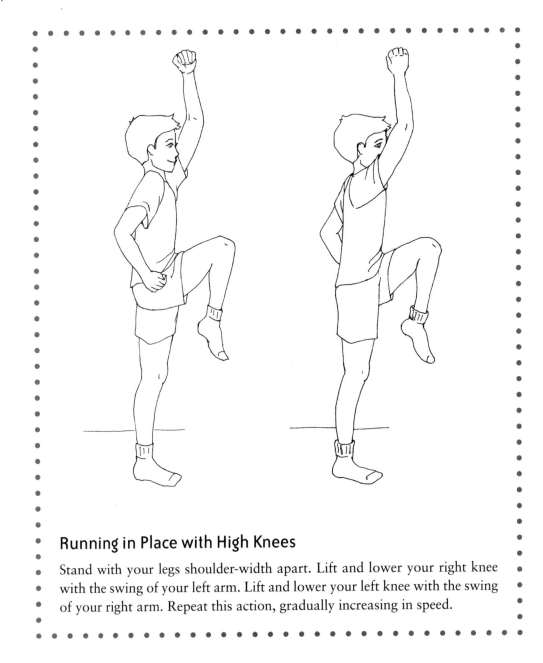

Running in Place with High Knees

Stand with your legs shoulder-width apart. Lift and lower your right knee with the swing of your left arm. Lift and lower your left knee with the swing of your right arm. Repeat this action, gradually increasing in speed.

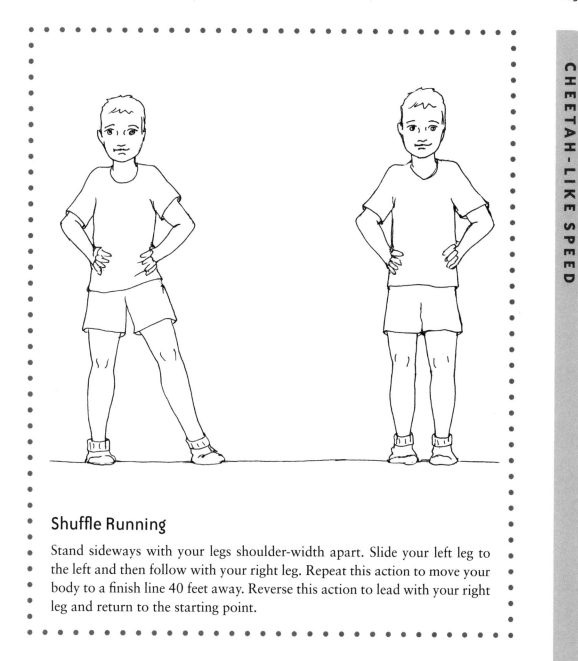

Shuffle Running

Stand sideways with your legs shoulder-width apart. Slide your left leg to the left and then follow with your right leg. Repeat this action to move your body to a finish line 40 feet away. Reverse this action to lead with your right leg and return to the starting point.

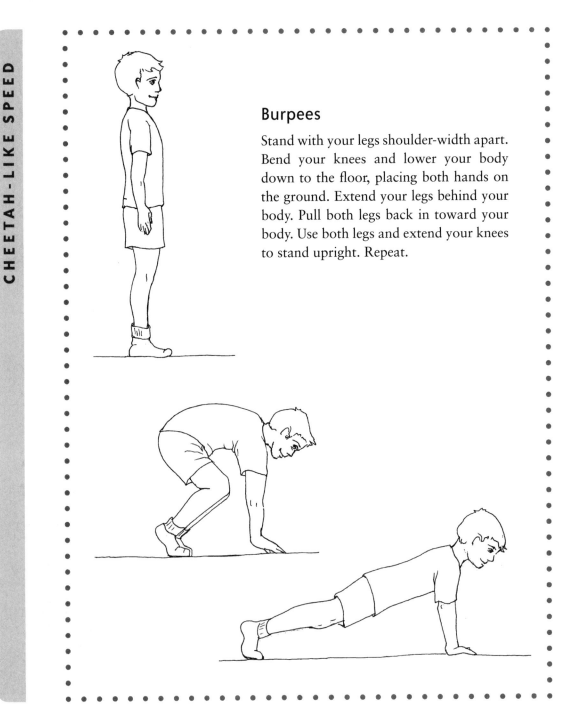

Burpees

Stand with your legs shoulder-width apart. Bend your knees and lower your body down to the floor, placing both hands on the ground. Extend your legs behind your body. Pull both legs back in toward your body. Use both legs and extend your knees to stand upright. Repeat.

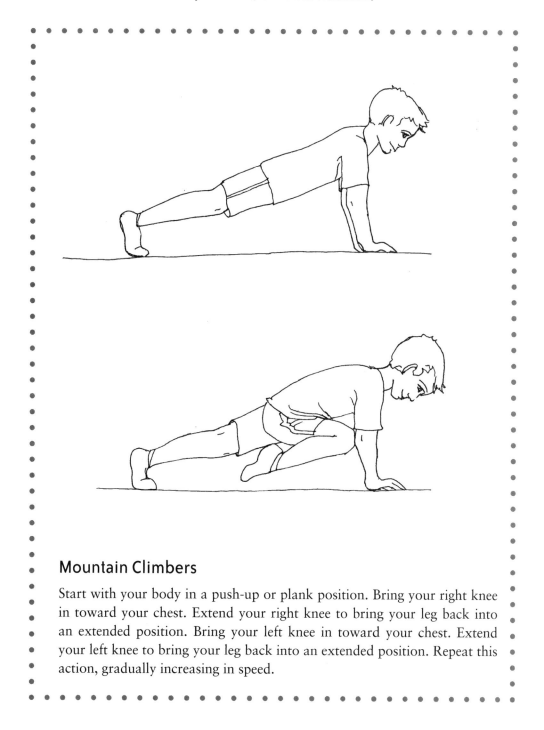

Mountain Climbers

Start with your body in a push-up or plank position. Bring your right knee in toward your chest. Extend your right knee to bring your leg back into an extended position. Bring your left knee in toward your chest. Extend your left knee to bring your leg back into an extended position. Repeat this action, gradually increasing in speed.

CAT-LIKE FLEXIBILITY

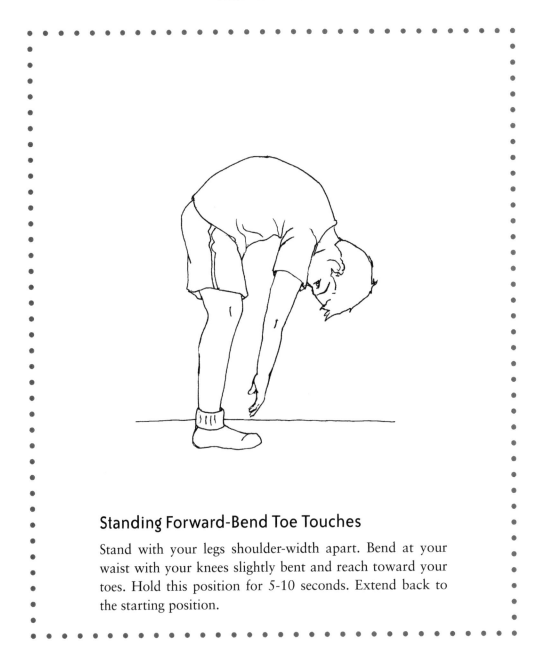

Standing Forward-Bend Toe Touches

Stand with your legs shoulder-width apart. Bend at your waist with your knees slightly bent and reach toward your toes. Hold this position for 5-10 seconds. Extend back to the starting position.

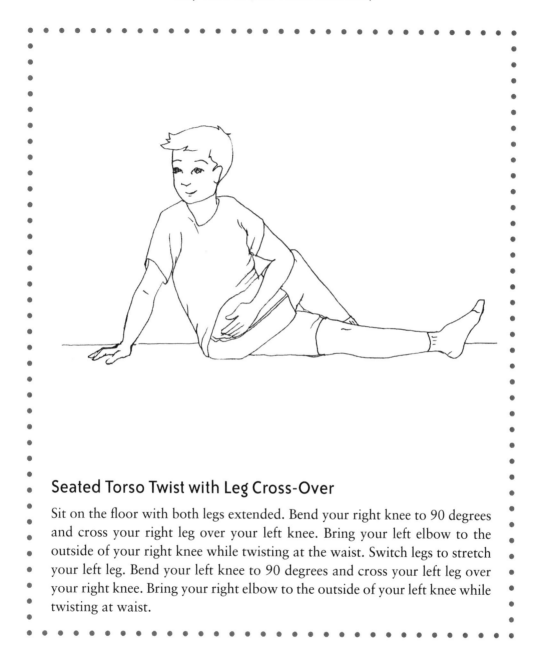

Seated Torso Twist with Leg Cross-Over

Sit on the floor with both legs extended. Bend your right knee to 90 degrees and cross your right leg over your left knee. Bring your left elbow to the outside of your right knee while twisting at the waist. Switch legs to stretch your left leg. Bend your left knee to 90 degrees and cross your left leg over your right knee. Bring your right elbow to the outside of your left knee while twisting at waist.

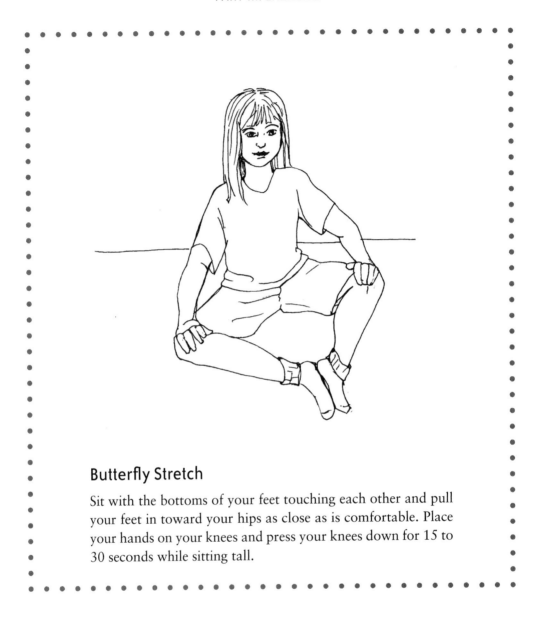

Butterfly Stretch

Sit with the bottoms of your feet touching each other and pull your feet in toward your hips as close as is comfortable. Place your hands on your knees and press your knees down for 15 to 30 seconds while sitting tall.

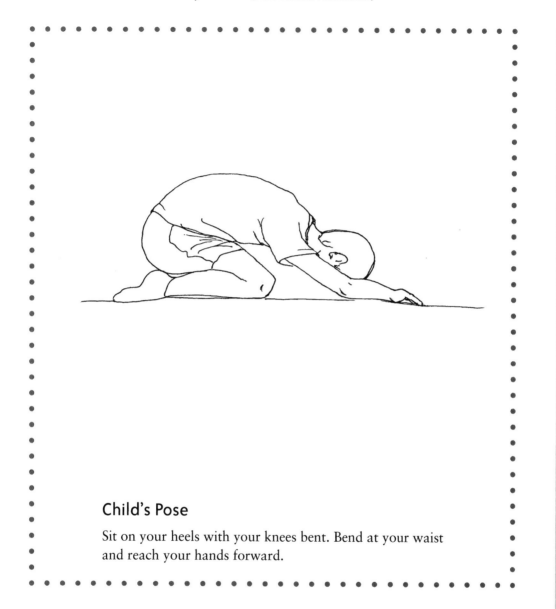

Child's Pose

Sit on your heels with your knees bent. Bend at your waist and reach your hands forward.

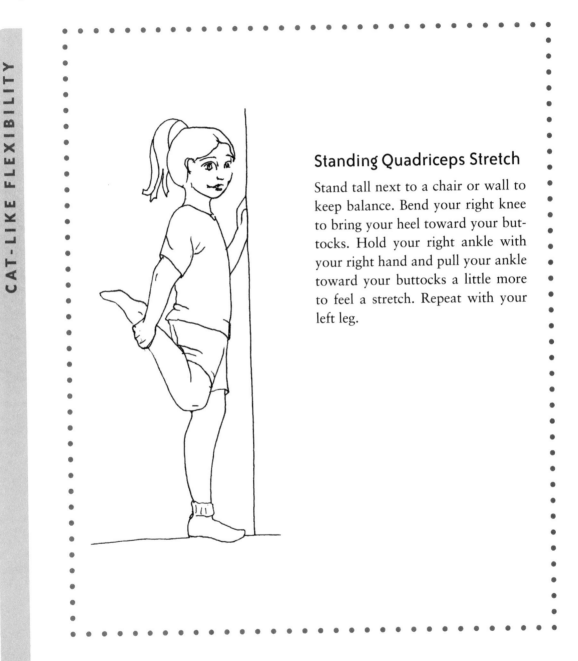

Standing Quadriceps Stretch

Stand tall next to a chair or wall to keep balance. Bend your right knee to bring your heel toward your buttocks. Hold your right ankle with your right hand and pull your ankle toward your buttocks a little more to feel a stretch. Repeat with your left leg.

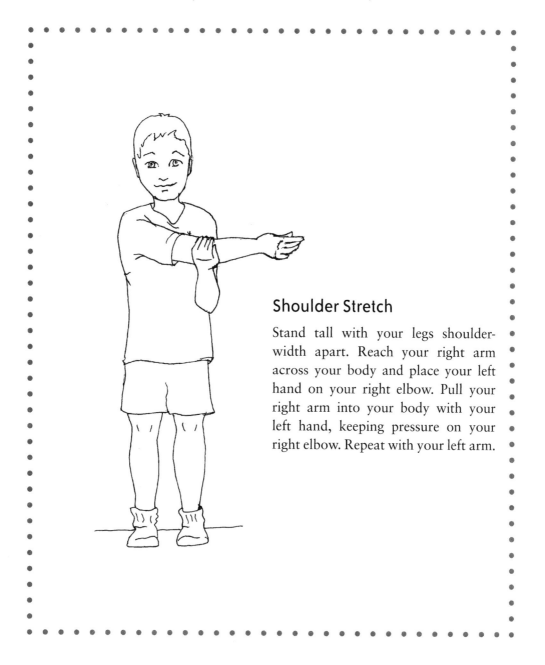

Shoulder Stretch

Stand tall with your legs shoulder-width apart. Reach your right arm across your body and place your left hand on your right elbow. Pull your right arm into your body with your left hand, keeping pressure on your right elbow. Repeat with your left arm.

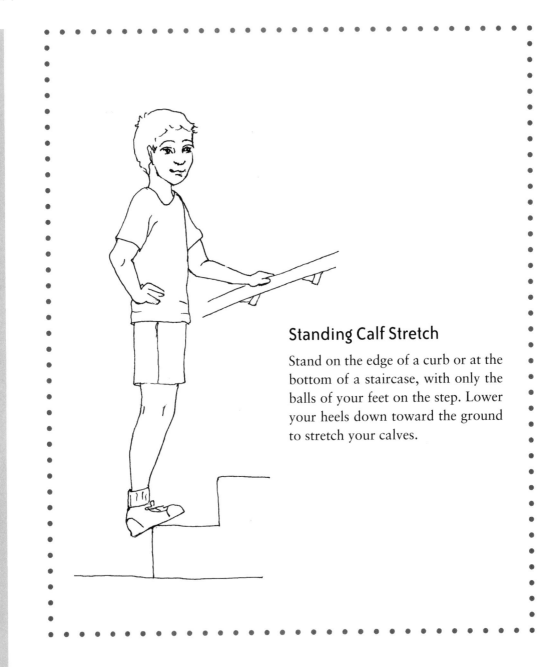

Standing Calf Stretch

Stand on the edge of a curb or at the bottom of a staircase, with only the balls of your feet on the step. Lower your heels down toward the ground to stretch your calves.

Chapter 8

GET OUT AND PLAY! • • • • • • • • • •
(Outdoor Recreational Activities)

O UTDOOR PLAY IS AN ideal way for kids to get the physical activity they need for healthy bodies and minds. Not only do they benefit from the exercise, they also get plenty of room to move freely and gain exposure to nature, fresh air, and sunlight.

The activities and games that can be enjoyed outdoors by you and your family are almost as limitless as the outdoors itself. In this chapter, you will find suggestions for some of our favorite activities to be enjoyed as individuals, with friends and family, or in larger groups.

> ## SAFETY FIRST!
>
> Your health *and* your safety are important to us. Always remember to protect your skin from the sun, wear the proper safety gear, and watch for cars and other hazards whenever you're outside enjoying outdoor sports and activities.

Tips from the top!

Bone-strengthening activities (such as tennis, basketball, and hopscotch) remain especially important for children and young adolescents because the greatest gains in bone mass occur during the years just before and during puberty. In addition, the majority of peak bone mass is obtained by the end of adolescence.

—*2008 Physical Activity Guidelines for Americans*, U.S. Department of Health and Human Services

INDIVIDUAL ACTIVITIES

Running

Running is a great physical activity that requires very little equipment or preparation to get started. Just tie up your sneakers and go! You can run on your own (be sure to get permission from your parents, follow safety rules, and stay in safe areas), with friends or family, or as part of a running team with school. Consider getting involved and training for special walk/run events that are sponsored in your community. Not only will you get in shape, but you'll be helping raise money and awareness for worthy causes.

Biking

Riding bicycles the traditional way is fun, but if you're looking to make individual or group biking even more exciting and challenging, try this activity. Use plastic cones, hula hoops, or other common outdoor toys that you have in your garage to create a simple riding course through which to maneuver your bike. For newer or younger bike riders who are still learning the basics, simplify the riding course by drawing a chalk path and have them practice staying in between the lines and learning how to stop and start.

Jumping Rope

Jumping rope improves your reflexes, balance and coordination, bone density, and muscular endurance.

Try these fun variations with your jump rope to make things interesting, add multiple levels of intensity, and work your muscles in different ways:

* *Double Foot Bounce*: Jump off the ground about 2 inches, raising both feet at the same time and then landing with both feet together.

* *Single Foot Bounce*: Jump by alternating feet with each revolution of the rope. This jump is similar to the double foot bounce, except that only one foot leaves the ground with each rope rotation. This activity resembles a slow skip.

* *Jogging Step*: This variation adds more intensity to the activity by incorporating jogging with jumping rope. Start with a slow jog and then begin swinging the jump rope over your body. Each time the rope comes around your feet, skip over it while still maintaining a jog. Adjust the pace to add or reduce intensity.

* *High Step*: This jump is similar to the jogging step, but you add alternating high knee lifts to increase intensity.

* *Skier's Jump*: Begin with the double foot bounce. Then, while keeping your ankles close together, bounce from side to side while jumping the rope. It will resemble a zigzag skiing motion. Younger or less experienced jumpers might want to try this activity without the rope, and instead, stand with both feet on a line and jump back and forth over the line.

* *Jack Jumps*: Start with a double foot bounce and, once you're ready to begin the jumping jacks, spread your feet apart (about shoulder-width), and then bring them back together between each rope rotation. Keep the jumps fairly small to start with and then gradually do bigger jumps to make the activity more challenging.

Skateboarding and/or Inline Skating

While you can practice skateboarding and inline skating almost anywhere that has smooth skating surfaces, you might also want to scout out local skate parks in your area. They have built-in ramps, half-pipes, and other obstacles that make the sport more adventurous. You'll also find lots of opportunities to meet other kids who share the same interests. Just make sure you remember to obey the skate park rules, bring your own equipment, and wear all your protective gear!

Swimming

Swimming is a sport that gets you moving, cools you down while working you out, and can be enjoyed solo or with a group of friends or family. You can swim laps, practice treading water, or dive for objects. If you have a few friends or family at the pool with you, set up relay races or play your favorite water games, like water volleyball or water tag. Always follow water safety rules and make sure an adult or lifeguard is nearby when you're in the water.

ACTIVITIES WITH FRIENDS

Tag

Tag is a group activity that is fun and easy for kids of all ages to play. One child is chosen to be "it" and has to chase the others and touch (tag) them. When a player is tagged, she or he becomes the new "it."

Try one of these twists to change up your tag game:

* *Team Tag*: Instead of one child being "it," pair into teams of two and link arms with your partner. The "it" must then try to link arms with one member of the team. The other part of the team who "it" didn't link with then becomes the new "it." Kids must always stay linked with a partner unless they are "it."

* *Reverse Tag*: Reverse tag is played much like traditional tag, but the object is reversed. An "it" is chosen, and all the other players count to ten while "it" runs away. All of the players then try to tag "it," instead of "it" doing the tagging. The child that tags "it" will then become the new "it" who must be tagged.

Two-Square or Four-Square

To play four-square, you will need a section of concrete or blacktop, a piece of chalk, a rubber playground ball (or volleyball), and at least four players. Begin by drawing a large 6 foot wide square. Divide that square into four smaller, equal squares and then number them 1 through 4.

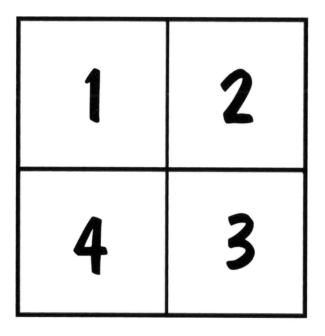

One player stands in each of the four squares. The player in square four serves the ball and tries to hit it into one of the other squares. The child in the receiving square must hit the ball into another player's square before it bounces twice. A player is out if she or he fails to hit the ball before the second bounce or if she or he misses another player's square. When someone gets out, the others move up one square and that player moves to the last square—or to the end of the line if more than four children are playing. The object of the game is to move up to, and maintain, the server position.

Two-square is played the same way as four-square, except only two squares are used and a minimum of two children are needed.

Dodgeball

A traditional game of dodgeball is generally played against a wall or the side of a building, with all players but one lined up along the wall. The other child is the thrower and must throw rubber playground balls at the other players (below the neck) while they try to dodge the balls. The thrower receives a point for each child she or he hits. Kids take turns being the thrower after a predetermined amount of time, typically 2 to 3 minutes.

If there are more children playing, another variation is to break into two equal teams. Use a rope to make a center line and have each team line up on opposite sides of the line. Each team starts with a ball and must then try to hit players of the opposing team with it. If a player is hit, she or he is out and must leave the playing area and sit down for the remainder of the game. If a player catches the ball that's thrown at her or him, the person who threw the ball is out. The game ends when only one child remains.

Hide and Seek

Hide and Seek is similar to tag except that players hide from the person designated to be "it," who is called the "seeker." When a player is found, she or he must race to the predetermined home base before being tagged by the "seeker."

Try these fun variations:

* *Sardines*: Sardines is a backward version of the traditional hide-and-seek game. Only one child starts out as the "hider," and the rest of the group are the "seekers." The group counts to a predetermined number (40 or 50 works well) to give the child time to find a good hiding spot. When a "seeker" finds the "hider," they must then hide with her or him in the hiding spot. Eventually all of the "seekers" except for the last one will be hiding in the same hiding spot, packed in like sardines. A new game begins when the last "seeker" finds the entire group in the hiding spot.

* *Chain Hide and Seek*: This version starts with one child as "it" and all the others hiding. As each player is found and caught before returning to base, they must join hands with "it" and stay connected as they continue to seek and catch all the other players. The longer the chain grows, the harder it becomes to tag the remaining participants and the more laughter results.

Backwards Baseball

Playing baseball and running bases is an excellent way to get exercise outdoors. Instead of playing baseball the same old way every time, mix things up once in a while with this fun variation on a classic game. Players must run the bases clockwise instead of counter-clockwise. Once the batter hits the ball, she or he must first run to third, then second, then first, and finally, home again. To add an extra challenge for adults and older kids, try also reversing their batting stance and having them bat from the opposite side of home plate. For instance, if they are normally a "leftie," have them hit from the right side.

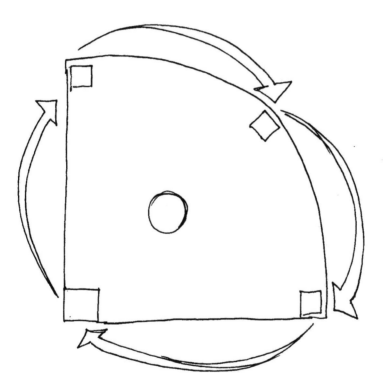

Basketball

In addition to playing a game of basketball with your friends, you can also get a good workout by playing shooting games and practicing passing drills on the court.

Here are a few fun variations to try with your friends:

* *Pass the Ball*: Perfect your passing skills by playing a game of Pass the Ball with your friends. Two players at a time sidestep down the basketball court while passing the ball back and forth. If more than two kids are playing, when a player loses control of the ball or misses the pass, she or he must sit out and the next child takes his or her place. Alternate the types of passes (such as the chest pass, bounce pass, baseball pass, and two-handed overhead pass) you use to improve your passing skills.

* *Shoot and Score*: Host contests to test your skills at dunking and shooting lay-ups and three-pointers. Playing a game of *Horse* with your friends is also a fun activity for the basketball court. One player first chooses the location and type of shot she or he wants to make. If the basket is made, all of the other players must shoot from the same spot. Any players that miss the shot must take the letter H, and so on until the word horse is spelled. She or he continues without a letter if the shot is made. The player with the least number of letters at the end of the game wins.

Soccer

Practice your soccer dribbling skills and ball handling by adding a soccer ball to the classic kids' game Red Light, Green Light. Have all the kids (except for one) start at one side of the field, each with a soccer ball. The child without a ball is the traffic cop and stands on the other side of the field. She or he yells "green light" and turns with his or her back to the others. The players must all start moving forward while dribbling their soccer balls. The traffic cop waits for a few moments, yells "red light," and turns back around. The players must stop and stand still with one foot on top of their soccer balls. Any child who gets caught still moving or who doesn't have his or her ball must return to the starting line.

Psst... Parents

The best way to get your kids interested in being active outdoors—and keep them motivated to exercise—is to get out there and be active with them. The "do as I say, not as I do" approach is not going to encourage your kids to be healthier and more active. No matter what age they are or what they may tell you, kids mimic what they see their parents doing. They need to see evidence that being healthy is a priority for you, too. Getting your family fit and staying that way requires teamwork and effort from the entire family. Plus, truthfully, spending time playing outdoors with your kids can be a lot of fun!

So what can you do with them outside? The majority of the activities that are listed above as suggestions for kids to do alone or with their friends can also be enjoyed with their parents, so take your cue from those ideas. Activities like participating in sports, playing catch with a ball or Frisbee, taking bike rides and runs together, and playing outdoor games are all excellent ways for parents and children to get exercise while spending quality time with each other.

Are you looking for an outdoor activity to enjoy as a family? Take a hike! Not only will you get fresh air and exercise together, but you'll also have plenty of opportunities to appreciate nature in the great outdoors and have important bonding time with your kids. Whether you're in the city or the country, there are parks, paths, and nature trails just waiting for you to explore them.

GROUP GAMES FOR SPECIAL EVENTS

Outdoor activities can also be an excellent addition to parties; neighborhood get-togethers; or church, school, or family events. Why limit fitness and fun to your own family circle? The great thing about exercise is that it doesn't have to always be structured or tedious in order to work. Let your imagination and sense of humor guide you when trying out these amusing games by tailoring them to fit your needs or creating your own activities.

Wacky Obstacle Course

Use whatever supplies (such as plastic cones, folding chairs, and jump ropes) you have in your home or garage to mark separate areas for your obstacle course. Each station should have a different activity to perform with a sign explaining the rules for that station. The number of stations and the complexity of the activities are up to you. For example, you can create a station where participants have to sit on a folding chair and use a stick (or baseball bat) to pretend they are rowing a boat while singing "Row, Row, Row Your Boat." Another station might instruct participants to jump rope 20 times and then run backwards to the next spot. The person with the fastest time wins, so be sure to have a paper, pen, and a stopwatch (or a watch with a second hand) available to time and record them.

The Wacky Obstacle Course can be tailored to whatever size group or family you have. Kids will get pleasure from competing and watching others complete the course. Hint: They especially love seeing their parents or teachers complete the course!

Get Ready, Get Dressed, and Go Relay Race

Get the group moving and laughing with a humorous twist on a relay race. This activity involves kids racing to dress in oversized clothes and accessories that they put over their own clothing and then running to a designated spot. To prepare for the relay race, you'll need to borrow some clothing items and accessories (like sunglasses, hats, and ties) from grownups' closets or purchase a few inexpensive ones from a thrift store. The bigger and funnier looking the items are the better!

Divide the kids into two teams and have each team line up single file. Set up the lawn chairs approximately 25 yards from the teams. Give the first players from each team a bag filled with the same amount of items (shorts, shirts, sunglasses, hats, necklace or necktie, etc.). When the game begins, the first players on each team must put on all the items in the bag, run down to the chair, return to their team, remove the items and place them back into the bag, then hand the bag to the next player in line. The relay continues until the whole team has participated. This game presents some hilarious photo opportunities, so be sure to have your camera ready!

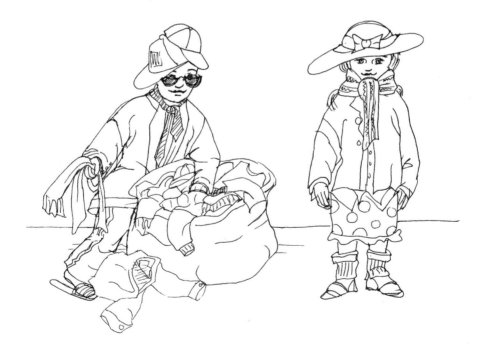

Wet and Wild Volleyball

Set up the volleyball net and get ready for a "Wet and Wild" version of this game. All you need is the volleyball net, a bunch of filled water balloons, two large bed sheets (or over-sized towels if it's a small group), and a group of players who are ready to get wet.

Divide the kids (and adults) into two teams. Line up the teams on either side of the net and give each team a bed sheet. All the members of the team must continue holding a section of the sheet at all times. Place a water balloon in the middle of the serving team's sheet. The players must work together to toss the water balloon over the net. The team on the other side must use their sheet to catch the water balloon. The volley continues until the balloon pops. The game continues until all the water balloons are gone and all the players are wet!

FAQS •

✳ **Our family is not used to exercising and eating healthy. Will Combat Fat for Kids! still be a plausible plan for us?** Yes! The program is designed with people from all backgrounds and levels of fitness in mind. The premise of our approach is not to make radical, impractical changes that families will have a hard time maintaining. Instead, the focus is on learning to make smart choices about exercise and nutrition. In the words of *Combat Fat* author Andrew Flach, "What you eat is what you get. We can choose to make better choices." The same principle applies to making decisions about physical fitness. You make the choices that best fit your family.

✳ **Does this mean I will have to cook separate meals for my kids and the adults in my house so that everyone gets what they like and need nutritionally?** No! The beauty of the recipes we've included is that they were selected with the needs and preferences of the whole family in mind. Not only will they work for everyone, most of them are created from ingredients that are typically stocked in most homes and can be found in your own backyard or local farmers' market. Remember: Don't be afraid to experiment with swapping out ingredients to please everyone's taste buds. Part of the fun in cooking as a family is that you get to try new things together!

✳ **My child is a very picky eater. Will this plan work for us?** It sure will! We, too, are parents of young children, so this issue was one that we took into consideration when planning the nutritional section of the book. Many of the recipes found in this book are healthier twists on favorites for most kids, like our Modified Macaroni 'n Cheese (see page 75). We've also addressed the issue of dealing with picky eaters and junk food lovers in Chapter 2: Common Challenges to Staying Fit as a Family (see page 20).

★ **We were doing well for awhile with the *Combat Fat for Kids!* program, and then we hit a bump and gave up. Now what?** Call a family meeting to identify the stumbling blocks your family encountered and determine how to overcome them or work around them. Then brush yourselves off and get back on the program! The *Combat Fat for Kids!* approach is about making smart choices every day, not about attaining perfection.

★ **My child does not look obese or overweight. How can I know for sure if she or he falls in a healthy range?** Being obese or overweight doesn't have just one look. It is possible for a child's body to carry excess fat or weight (or both) without his or her body necessarily looking like it. The best way to identify your child's body fat measurements and to learn where she or he falls on the weight scale for a particular height and age is to visit your family physician. Be proactive and request that your child's physician perform health screenings and health assessments (like skinfold thickness measurements) and examine family history and your child's current diet and activity level.

★ **How long does it take to complete the *Combat Fat for Kids!* plan?** In a word . . . forever. Now don't get scared! A healthy lifestyle should always require a lifetime commitment. *Combat Fat for Kids!* is not designed to be a quick fix or fad diet and exercise plan that gets kids and families in shape and then lets them loose to return to their previous way of eating and exercising. Instead, our goal is to teach you and your children basic methods that can be used, altered, and applied to the rest of your life. Our aim is to get your family healthy and teach them how to stay that way.

★ **My family members have very hectic schedules. How well will the *Combat Fat for Kids!* plan fit into our already busy lifestyle?** We understand that most families today have busy schedules to juggle. There is no need for long hours of preparation and implantation to reap the benefits of the program. That's why the book is full of time-saving suggestions and ways to make small changes that you can implement over time to bring about huge positive results.

★ **What about during holidays or when we're on a family vacation? How can we still make the *Combat Fat for Kids!* plan a priority?** There is a huge misconception that it's impossible to eat healthy and stay active during the holidays. We disagree! In fact, vacations and holidays often lend extra together time for families to incorporate some fun activities into their day. You simply have to look for them. Are you camping out with your family and friends or maybe hosting a holiday get-together? Get your family and friends involved in the action. Check out the Outdoor Recreation Activities listed in Chapter 8 and alter it to fit your group.

We guarantee that eating healthy can be included in your vacation or holiday, too! Remember, the key to success is to make wiser choices in what you eat and drink. Maintaining proper portion control, making healthy substitutions, and enjoying special treats in moderation can keep you and your whole family on track. Don't forget that we have also included a large section of healthy and tasty recipes in this book that can be included in your holiday celebrations, such as the Cornbread-Crusted Turkey (see page 100), Cucumber Yogurt Dip (see page 106), and Black Bean Brownies (see page 112).

★ **Our family has kids of varying age ranges. Can *Combat Fat for Kids!* work for all of them?** Yes, it can and does. The driving factor behind the *Combat Fat for Kids!* plan is to help your kids and family find a healthy balance in nutrition and physical activity. The ideas mentioned in the book are simply a starting point to get families thinking about how to make positive changes, not the end-all. Feel free to alter the program to fit the needs of your entire family. If your young child has an aversion to certain foods, it is perfectly fine to make healthy substitutions to the recipes to make them more appealing. If an exercise or game in this book seems too easy for your teenager, add an extra boost to the activity to make it more challenging.

★ **My kid is a teenager. Any suggestions on how I can motivate her or him to get involved with the *Combat Fat for Kids!* program?** Kids in this age group may be more distracted by technology, friends, and busy schedules. Our best advice is to be honest and direct with your teenager about the need for finding a healthy balance in his or her diet, activity level, and overall lifestyle. Teens are mature enough to understand reason when it's presented in a loving, non-accusatory way. Of course, after you talk, action is also necessary. Get your teen involved in the family planning. Allow her or him to help in deciding and preparing meals. Put your teenager in charge of selecting the type of family activity or exercise for certain days of the week. In order for kids—especially those who are learning to make their own decisions—to be excited about making changes, they must feel ownership in it. Getting older kids involved in the decision and implementation process not only ensures that they will enjoy the chosen foods and activities more, it also prepares them for the future by teaching them valuable skills that will help them maintain a healthy life into adulthood.

RESURCES · · · · · · · · · · · · · · · · · · ·

★ American Academy of Pediatrics (AAP)
  www.aap.org

★ American Heart Association (AHA)
  www.heart.org

★ American Institute for Cancer Research (AICR)
  www.aicr.org

★ Centers for Disease Control and Prevention (CDC)
  www.cdc.gov

★ ChooseMyPlate.gov from the United State Department of Agriculture (USDA)
  www.choosemyplate.gov

★ Combat Fat for Kids!
  www.combatfatforkids.com

★ Fruits & Veggies—More Matters from Produce for Better Health Foundation
  (PBH) www.FruitAandVeggiesMoreMatters.org

★ Health.gov
  www.health.gov

★ Healthy Schools Campaign (HSC)
  www.healthyschoolscampaign.org

★ The Jump Rope Institute
  www.jumpropeinstitute.com

* KidsHealth
  www.kidshealth.org

* Kids Running from Runner's World
  www.kidsrunning.com

* Let's Move!
  www.letsmove.gov

* National Eating Disorders Association (NEDA)
  www.nationaleatingdisorders.org
  (800) 931-2237

* National Heart, Lung, and Blood Institute (NHLBI)
  www.nhlbi.nih.gov

* National Institute of Child Health and Human Development
  (NICHD)
  www.nichd.nih.gov

* National Institute of Mental Health (NIMH)
  www.nimh.nih.gov

* United States Department of Agriculture (USDA)
  www.usda.gov

* USDA Meat and Poultry Hotline
  1-888-MPHotline
  1-888-674-6854

* United States Department of Health and Human Services (HHS)
  www.hhs.gov

ABOUT THE AUTHORS · · · · · · · · · · ·

JAMES VILLEPIGUE, a father of three and best-selling author of the *Body Sculpting Bible* series, has over 20 years of experience in the health and fitness industry as a nationally certified personal trainer with The National Strength & Conditioning Association (NSCA), with their prestigious Certified Strength & Conditioning Specialist (CSCS) credential, The American Council on Exercise and The International Sports Science Association. He has received degrees from Hofstra University, the New York College of Health Professions, and the Institute for Professional Empowerment Coaching. He now lives in East North Port, New York.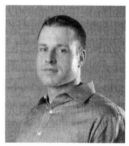

JO BRIELYN is an author and contributing writer for Hatherleigh Press and has currently completed 13 nonfiction books about health and wellness. Jo is an author and poet whose works have appeared in three Twin Trinity Media anthologies: *Elements of the Soul, Elements of Time,* and *Elements of Life.* Jo is the founder, writer, and editor of Creative Kids Ideas, a resource website that supplies parents, teachers, and family members with the tips and fun ideas to help build stronger, happier, and more creative kids. She is also a devoted mom and wife, former youth leader, and veteran of the United States Air Force. Jo resides in Central Florida with her husband and their two daughters.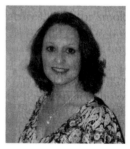

Notes